Basic Biomechanics Explained

Titles in the series
Basic Biomechanics Explained
Electrotherapy Explained
Human Movement Explained
Physical Principles Explained

Basic Biomechanics Explained

John Low BA(Hons), FCSP, DipTP, SRP

Formerly Acting Principal, School of Physiotherapy, Guy's Hospital, London, UK

Ann Reed BA, MCSP, DipTP, SRP

Senior Lecturer, Department of Health Studies, University of East London, UK

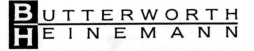

Butterworth-Heinemann
Linacre House, Jordan Hill, Oxford OX2 8DP
A division of Reed Educational and Professional Publishing Ltd

ℛ A member of the Reed Elsevier plc group

OXFORD   BOSTON   JOHANNESBURG
MELBOURNE   NEW DELHI   SINGAPORE

First published 1996
Reprinted 1997

British Library Cataloguing in Publication Data
A catalogue record for this book is available from the British Library

Library of Congress Cataloguing in Publication Data

A catalogue record for this book is available from the Library of Congress

Library of Congress Cataloguing in Publication Data

A catalogue record for this book is available from the Library of Congress

ISBN 0 7506 2103 6

Typeset by Bath Typesetting Ltd
Printed and bound in Great Britain by Hartnolls Ltd, Bodmin, Cornwall

Contents

Preface

This book is intended as an introduction to some of the biomechanical material and concepts forming a necessary foundation for the study of physiotherapy and other health sciences. It is also hoped that it may be useful to graduate therapists.

In attempting to describe and explain at an introductory level, we have presumed no advanced level familiarity with any basic subjects except some anatomy and physiology. The material covered is wide ranging so that many aspects of biomechanics have been introduced. Where appropriate, we have involved clinical applications, both to illustrate biomechanical principles and to provide information of practical usefulness.

We are indebted in this work to students and colleagues for their advice, to our families and friends for their tolerance, and to Caroline Makepeace and her colleagues at Butterworth-Heinemann for their customary support and good humour.

John Low
Ann Reed

POSTSCRIPT FROM A. R.

Those of you who know me may be surprised that I am putting my name, albeit as a co-author, to a book on biomechanics. The fact is that this is John's work, but, because we have established such a great working rapport from our previous two books, he asked me to continue our partnership with the third in the trilogy. From this you will gather that if you like the book it will be due to my editorial hand, but if you find fault with it I am afraid I must refer you to John!

A.R.

1.   *Biomechanics: force and energy*

Biomechanics refers to the mechanics of movements in living creatures, particularly, in this book, in humans. It is a branch of biophysics that combines biology, physiology, physics, engineering and medicine. Since mechanics is the science dealing with the behaviour of matter under the action of force, these are the two principal subjects of the first two chapters.

DEVELOPMENT OF BIOMECHANICS

Biomechanics is a young discipline and as such is often only vaguely defined. It shares many areas with older disciplines. Thus, a very brief look at the way it has developed may be helpful.

Giovanni Borelli (1608–1679) is often considered the 'father of biomechanics', since he clearly attempted to integrate physiology and physical science in his 1680 publication *De motu animalum*. He described human and animal movement, including human gait analysis, in mechanical terms and offered thoughts on the function of muscles, the direction of their fibres, fatigue and pain. This work was being done in the context of the seventeenth century revolution in scientific thinking, so that the study of biomechanics could go forward on the basis of the fundamental work of Galileo Galilei (1564–1642), Johannes Kepler (1571–1630), Renee Descartes (1596–1650) and Isaac Newton (1642–1727), which culminated in a new understanding of mechanics and mathematics, the mechanics being synthesized in 'Newton's laws'. Others whose work at this time formed the basis of biomechanics included Robert Hooke (see Chapter 2), William Harvey (1561–1636), whose explanation of the circulation of the blood is well known, and Borelli himself, as well as numerous others. The invention of the light microscope greatly aided the study of physiology in the latter part of this period.

However, it should not be thought that there had been no interest in biomechanics prior to the seventeenth century. Galen (AD 131–201), whose writings and beliefs dominated medical science for some 1300 years, apparently had a life-long interest in the mechanism of movement. In particular, the role of the muscles that he described in *De motu musculorum* (*On the movements of muscles*) introduced such concepts as muscle contraction, muscle tone and the distinction between agonist and antagonist muscles. Prior to the Roman era, Greek civilization had produced the early scientists and great philosophers. Aristotle (384–322 BC), who was perhaps the greatest, provided a treatise *About the movement of animals*. In this he described movement, including a description of gait, with some analysis, and anticipated Newton's third law in noting ground reaction forces.

The Italian Renaissance of the fifteenth and early sixteenth centuries provided some scientific activity, notably in anatomical studies, after nearly 13 centuries in which little had been published since Galen. The anatomical and mechanical drawings of Leonardo da Vinci (1452–1579) are well known, whilst Vesalius (1514–1564) redefined the anatomy of Galen and provided a modern view of muscle action.

Since Borelli in the seventeenth century, there has been an almost continuous expansion of understanding in biomechanics, especially in mathematics and muscle physiology. The 'enlightenment' of the eighteenth century was a period of very intense scientific work. The development of new technologies during the nineteenth century encouraged the further study of motion. Amongst these, the invention of photography played a prominent part and enabled a more detailed study of locomotion, both human and animal. The pioneer of quantifying locomotion was Etienne Jules Marey (1838–1904), who developed numerous measuring devices and cine photography. He developed what must be regarded as the first 'gait laboratory' as the 'Station Physiologue' in the Parc des Princes, Paris (presently the Roland Garros tennis courts). Also at this time some understanding of electricity was developing, which led to the use of electrical stimulation and electromyography. The present century has seen further rapid technical development allowing still more precise measurement and extending visualization, notably by the development of the electron microscope, which influenced the understanding of mechanical changes at a cellular level. The possibility of radical replacement surgery has prompted the detailed study of the behaviour of materials within the body when under load. It has also seen the development of biomechanics as an academic subject and the separate development of related disciplines such as ergonomics (see Chapter 11).

For an account of the historical highlights on the path to modern biomechanics, see Nigg (1994). It seems likely that further advances in biomechanics will be seen in the future to have been due to the ability of the computer to handle large quantities of data.

MATTER AND MOTION

The physical world may be described in terms of matter and energy. The former occupies space and has mass, while the latter is the capacity of a system to do work. It is necessary to have a means of describing both matter and motion by some universally agreed method.

There are three fundamental concepts, measured in internationally agreed units, from which many others can be derived:

1. The concept of length or distance, measured in metres.
2. The concept of amount or quantity of matter, measured in kilograms.

3. The concept of time, measured in seconds.

From these fundamental dimensions many other units can be derived. For example:

Length × length = area in square metres, e.g. $2\,m \times 2\,m = 4\,m^2$

$$\text{Length} \times \text{length} \times \text{length} = \text{volume in cubic metres},$$
$$\text{e.g. } 2\,m \times 2\,m \times 2\,m = 8\,m^3$$

$$\frac{\text{Mass}}{\text{Volume}} = \text{density, e.g. } \frac{16\,kg}{8\,m^3} = 2\ kg\ m^{-3}$$

N.B. (The notation $2\,kg\,m^{-3}$ means 2 kilograms per cubic metre. Similarly, $2\,m\,s^{-1}$ means 2 metres per second. This form will be used throughout.)

$$\frac{\text{Distance}}{\text{Time}} = \text{speed, measured in metres per second, e.g. m } s^{-1}$$

$$\frac{\text{Distance in a uniform direction}}{\text{Time}} = \text{velocity, measured in m } s^{-1}$$

$$\frac{\text{Distance}}{\text{Time} \times \text{time}} = \text{acceleration, measured in m } s^{-2}$$

While the first three examples describe matter, the next three are concerned with motion and lead to a most important concept – that of force.

FORCE

Force is that which alters or tends to alter the state of motion of a body. In simple terms, forces are pushes and pulls. The idea of force is central to what is to follow in connection with stress or pressure, body movement and much else.

Newton's first law of motion tells us that a force is needed to alter the velocity of a body, i.e. to change its speed or direction of motion. This means that if a body is stationary the forces acting upon it must be balanced with one another and the system is said to be in equilibrium. If the body is moving it will continue to move at a constant speed until a force causes it to stop, slow down, speed up or change direction.

Moving bodies possess a quantity of motion called *momentum*. It is equal to the mass times the velocity of the body (*mv*).

Newton's second law of motion explains that the rate of change of momentum of a given body is proportional to the resultant force acting upon it and takes place in the direction of the force.

This is simply an extension of the first law and means that, for example, a large force acting on a small object will accelerate it rapidly (say, a hefty kick of a light ball) whereas a small force acting on a large object will accelerate it slowly.

Rate of change of momentum can be written as mass (m) times acceleration (a). Expressed in symbols, this is:

$$F = ma$$

Force (F) is measured in *newtons* (N). The force needed to accelerate a body of 1 kg mass at $1\,\mathrm{m\,s}^{-2}$ is 1 N. If a force is applied to a 1 kg object such that at the end of 1 second the object has a velocity of $1\,\mathrm{m\,s}^{-1}$ and at the end of the next second it has a velocity of $2\,\mathrm{m\,s}^{-1}$, and so on, then that force is 1 N. Similarly, a 1 kg object decelerating at $1\,\mathrm{m\,s}^{-2}$ would exert a force of 1 N.

$$N = \mathrm{kg\ m\,s}^{-2}$$

Notice that force, like velocity, is a *vector quantity*, which means it has *direction* as well as magnitude. Furthermore, force is not limited to objects physically connected to one another, like the foot kicking a ball, but includes forces that may act at a distance without physical contact, such as gravitational or magnetic forces.

Movements of the human body result from the motion of one body segment on another, say, the forearm and hand on the arm. (Body segments are described in Chapter 3.) Both segments will remain at rest until some force, say, the elbow flexor muscles, acts to overcome the inertia of the segment, setting, in this case, the hand and forearm in motion. This movement would continue until some other force, an opposing muscle pull or the tension of soft tissues for example, acts to overcome the inertia of the movement, thus bringing the part to rest. If the movement were to be performed more rapidly it would need a larger force, i.e. stronger muscle contraction. Likewise, if a weighty object were held in the hand, greater force would be needed. This example should raise many questions, such as how the muscle generates force and what part the numerous other forces acting on the body would play. Some of these questions will be considered in subsequent chapters.

Describing forces

To describe fully a force at one instance involves more than its magnitude. The line of action, direction and point of application are all pertinent. These features are often represented in force diagrams by the use of an arrow. The length of the arrow is drawn in proportion to the magnitude of the force in newtons, the shaft represents the line of action, and the head

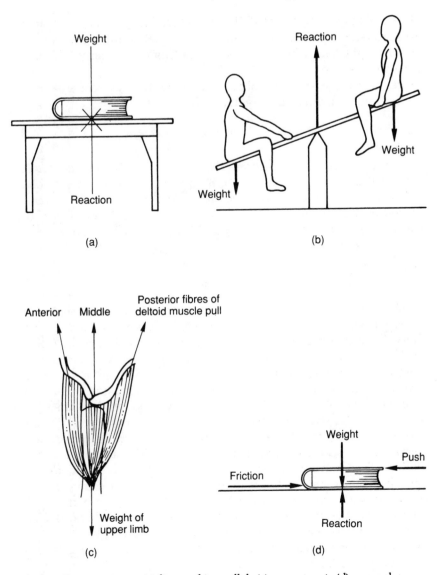

Fig. 1.1 Force systems: (a) linear; (b) parallel; (c) concurrent; (d) general.

shows the direction of the force. The position of the arrow with respect to objects or other forces shows the point of application. Diagrams are often drawn to illustrate force systems using such descriptive arrows (see, for example Figs 1.1–1.3). Such force diagrams are a valuable way of calculating resulting forces as well as illustrating force systems. In the latter case, the magnitude of the forces may be given only approximately or as a number beside the arrow.

Force systems may be divided and classified in various ways. *Static force systems*, in which the forces balance and there is no motion, can be

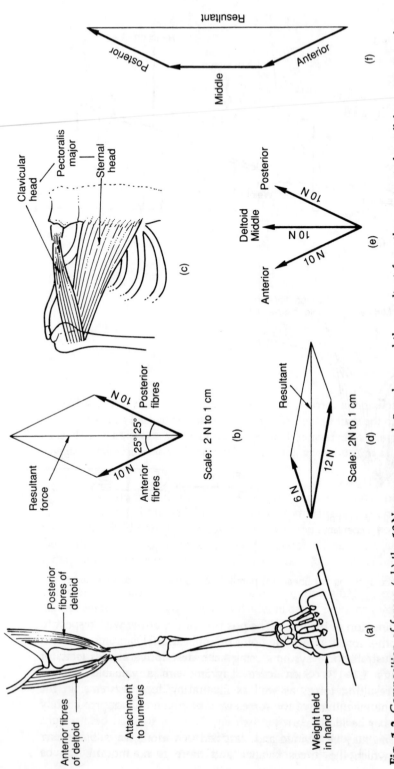

Fig. 1.2 Composition of forces; (a,b) the 10N arrows are each 5 cm long and the resultant from the constructed parallelogram is 9 cm long, hence the combined force is 18 N; (c,d.) the two force arrows of 3 cm and 6 cm lengths at an angle of 30° form a parallelogram whose diagonal is approximately 8.7 cm long, hence the combined force is 17.4 N; (e,f.) the three groups of fibres, each represented by a 5 cm arrow, form a polygon whose resultant completed side is 14 cm long, hence the combined force is 28 N.

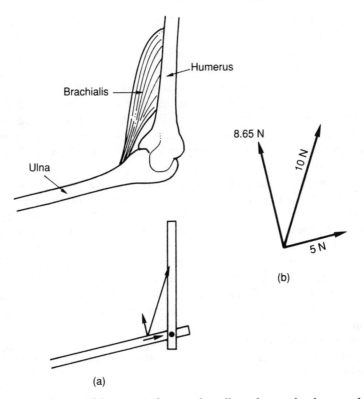

Fig. 1.3 Resolution of forces: (a) the muscle pull can be resolved into a force at right angles to the shaft of the ulna acting to flex the elbow and a force along the shaft causing joint compression; (b) if the muscle force is assumed to be 10 N at an angle of 60° to the horizontal, the other forces will be approximately as shown.

distinguished from *dynamic force systems* in which motion occurs. The former describes the system at a moment in time during which it is in equilibrium or balance. They are much used to describe body mechanics and are usually planar, i.e. forces acting in one plane only are considered. The latter involve velocity and other changes over time and are inevitably more complex.

Static force systems acting in one plane can be further conveniently subdivided by grouping those in which one or two of the variables remain constant:

1. *Linear force systems* are those in which the lines of action and points of application of the forces are constant, while the magnitude and direction are variable. These are pressure and tension systems such as a weight pressing down on a surface: a person standing on a floor or a book resting on a table, for example (see Fig. 1.1a); or it could be a weight hanging down in tension from a support, such as a light bulb hanging from the ceiling by a flex or the tension of the rope in a tug-of-war. Such

systems are further discussed in Chapter 2 and in connection with pressure in Chapter 8.

2. *Parallel force systems* are those in which only the lines of the forces are constant, while the magnitude, point of application and direction of the forces vary. Such systems are often concerned with rotation or torque, of which see-saws, cog wheels and simple lever systems are the usual cited examples (see Fig. 1.1b). Due to the fact that many joints in the human body exhibit approximately angular motion, there are numerous examples of parallel force systems in biomechanics, which are discussed in Chapter 5.

3. *Concurrent force systems* are those in which only the point of application is constant. The resulting force is a consequence of the magnitudes, directions and lines of action of the component forces, for example, two different groups of muscle fibres pulling at the same point on a bone, for example, the anterior and posterior fibres of the deltoid muscle (see Fig. 1.1c). This reinforces the point that forces are vector quantities; that is, they have both magnitude and direction. Thus, to define a particular force both must be given. This is in contradistinction to scalar quantities, which are fully described in terms of the appropriate units of magnitude, like temperature given in degrees Celsius.

4. Systems in which none of the variables are constant are known as *general force systems*. An example, shown in Figure 1.1d, is of a thick book being pushed along a surface.

Analysis of some simple force systems

Linear force systems in equilibrium will exhibit forces of equal and opposite magnitude. Thus, the book resting on the table in Figure 1.1a is pressing down due to the force of gravity acting on its mass (see Chapter 3) and the table is pressing up (see Chapter 2) a force of reaction. Thus, in a simple force diagram of this situation, the arrows representing the forces would be of equal length. Similarly, if a second book of the same weight were piled on top of the first, then both forces would be doubled, represented by arrows of twice the length.

Consider a concurrent force system in which two forces act at a point in two different directions. An example of this is the contribution to stabilizing the glenohumeral joint that the anterior and posterior fibres of deltoid make when the upper limb is dependent at the side with a weight in the hand (see Fig. 1.2a). If it is assumed that the average line of pull of the anterior fibres makes an angle of 50° with that of the posterior fibres, and that both sets of fibres pull equally with a force of 10 N, they would each support a weight of approximately 1 kg (acceleration due to gravity is $9.81\,\mathrm{m\,s^{-2}}$, therefore 1 kg exerts a force of 9.81 N). The combined effect of these two forces is not a matter of simple addition but can be found by drawing a parallelogram to scale and measuring the diagonal, which is the resultant force (see Fig. 1.2b). The same reasoning can be applied to the assumed different forces exerted by the pectoral and clavicular heads of pectoralis major as shown in Figure 1.2c,d. In all these cases, the result can be found either by trigonometry or algebraically by the use of the Pythagoras theorem (see Appendix B).

If more than two forces are being considered, it is often simpler to use the polygon method. If the contribution of the middle fibres of the deltoid muscle is added into Figure 1.2a, the force diagram Figure 1.2e is produced, which may be converted to a polygon by drawing the arrows to scale (starting anywhere) and with the same orientation. Closing the polygon will give the resultant force from the length and direction of this final arrow (Fig. 1.2f).

These ways of finding the single force resulting from two or more other forces are referred to as *the composition of forces*. An opposite process, in which a single force can be divided into two or more component forces, is known as *the resolution of forces*. This can be shown by reversing the parallelogram method considered above. It is often useful to resolve the single diagonal force into vertical and horizontal components. An important example is of a muscle pulling at an angle on the shaft of a bone, as illustrated in Figure 1.3a. Part of the force is exerted at right angles to the shaft causing angular motion at the joint (see Chapter 5). The rest of the force acts along the shaft to cause compression at the joint. The magnitude of these two forces can be found by constructing a parallelogram as shown in Figure 1.3b. Naturally, these resolved forces do not simply summate to the original 10 N because they are proportional to their squares, i.e. $8.66^2 + 5^2 = 10^2$ (see Appendix B).

SYSTEMS OF MEASUREMENT

For dealing with and communicating about the physical world, systems of measurement are necessary. There are three aspects of measurement: the numerical value, the unit and the level of accuracy. For example, a piece of cloth might be described as 2.5 m long to the nearest cm.

The fundamental units of length, mass and time are entirely arbitrary, being chosen from a variety of human-sized measures which developed from practical use. Some of the names used in the old imperial system — feet and stones — make this very evident. The basic units are those that can be conveniently handled by humans. Thus a kilogram is the sort of mass that is often held in the hand and a metre is approximately the distance from one shoulder to the opposite outstretched hand, a posture often seen in unravelling a bolt of cloth or roughly measuring a length of flex. A second is approximately the interval between the beats of the resting human heart rate.

Actually the human body was widely used as a convenient yardstick during recorded history. The distance from the tip to the interphalangeal joint of the thumb is well known as the basis of the inch, but palms, fingers and cubits (olecranon to tip of long finger) were also used.

Four fingerwidths = 1 palm

Four palms = 1 foot = 36 barleycorns 'taken from the middle of the ear'

Six palms = 1 cubit

The yard, the distance from the tip of King Edgar's nose to the end of his middle finger on his outstreched arm, was legalized as 'our yard of Winchester' by Henry I, the son of William the Conqueror. The mile was derived from the Roman military system, 1000 (*mille*) legionnaires' strides. This was actually 1618 yards but the imperial standard became 1760 yards to the mile (Ritchie-Calder, 1970).

Table 1.1 Some International System (SI) units

Quantity	Unit	Symbol
Fundamental units		
Length (distance)	metre	m
Mass	kilogram	kg
Time	second	s
Other basic units		
Luminous intensity	candela	cd
Amount of substance	mole	mol
Temperature	kelvin	K
Electric current	ampere	A
Some derived units		
Electric charge	coulomb	C
Electric potential	volt	V
Electric resistance	ohm	Ω
Electric capacitance	farad	F
Inductance	henry	H
Magnetic flux density	tesla	T
Force	newton	N
Energy	joule	J
Power	watt	W
Frequency	hertz	Hz
Temperature	Celsius	°C
Pressure	pascal	Pa

The metre and kilogram were originally chosen by a French committee in 1791. The metre was arbitrarily taken as one-40 000 000th of the circumference of the earth. A standard length was set with which other standard lengths could be compared. In the late nineteenth century it was a platinum-iridium bar but since 1960 the wavelength of the orange-red line in the spectrum of krypton 86 (an isotope of an inert gas) has been used as the standard.

The kilogram is defined by a platinum-iridium mass of that weight used to check other standards by comparisons made on very sensitive balances. One thousandth of a kilogram, 1 gram, is almost exactly the mass of 1 cubic centimetre of water at 4°C.

The basic unit of time is the second, which is one-sixtieth of a minute and one-3600th of an hour, which, unfortunately, are not decimal relationships. The oscillations of atomic systems are currently used to give accurate time measurement.

Table 1.1 gives a list of International System (SI) Units divided into the seven basic or fundamental units and most of the derived units. The derivation of force has been considered above and many of the others will be discussed in subsequent chapters.

It might be considered that a fundamental unit would be that of momentum but curiously no unit is assigned to this quantity. As already described, the rate of change of momentum, which is known as force, is measured in newtons ($N = kg\,m\,s^{-2}$). Similarly, velocity is a quantity derived from arbitrary units of length and time, given in metres per second without a special unit.

There are several ways of dealing with large or difficult numbers and units. First, in the interests of simplicity, a recognized abbreviation is used for the units (Table 1.1). Secondly, recognized universal prefixes are used to indicate the magnitude of the unit, e.g. calling one-100th m 1 centimetre (Table 1.2). A way of dealing with numbers, especially large numbers, is known as the power of 10 notation, in which $10^2 = 100$, $10^3 = 1000$, and so on. This is fully described in Appendix A.

The level of accuracy of a measurement is of considerable importance but varies according to the circumstance. In buying a piece of cloth, as in the example above, specifying the length to micrometre level would be absurd and impossible but such precision may well be required for a metal part in an aircraft instrument. Further, the absolute size of what is being measured may influence the level of accuracy required. For instance, a half-kilogram error in a weighing machine may be perfectly reasonable for weighing 50 kg adults, giving 1% error, but unacceptable for weighing 3.5 kg babies, for whom it would give a 14% error. In some circumstances the accuracy may be more fully expressed by giving the average or mean of several measurements and the extent to which they vary from this mean. The word *validity*, when used of a measurement, refers to how closely the measurement conforms to the real dimension being measured. *Reliability* refers in this context to how closely different measurements of the same dimension agree with one another. Notice that in many situations reasonable reliability is required rather than validity. For example, in recording day-to-day changes in weight in the 3.5 kg baby considered above, what may be of importance is the *change* in weight.

Basic Biomechanics Explained

Providing, therefore, that the machine gives a repeatable reading from day to day and the same machine can always be used, the absolute weight may not be of consequence.

For the rest of this book, units will be given by their proper abbreviations according to the SI system (Tables 1.1 and 1.2).

Table 1.2 Prefixes for SI units

Prefix	Abbreviation	Multiplied factor	Function
tera	T	1 000 000 000 000	10^{12}
giga	G	1 000 000 000	10^{9}
mega	M	1 000 000	10^{6}
kilo	k	1000	10^{3}
hecto	h	100	10^{2}
deca	da	10	10^{1}
deci	d	0.1	10^{-1}
centi	c	0.01	10^{-2}
milli	m	0.001	10^{-3}
micro	μ	0.000 001	10^{-6}
nano	n	0.000 000 001	10^{-9}
pico	p	0.000 000 000 001	10^{-12}
femto	f	0.000 000 000 000 001	10^{-15}
atto	a	0.000 000 000 000 000 001	10^{-18}

ENERGY

To describe energy it is first necessary to consider energy changes, conversion of one form of energy to another. For example, electrical energy is converted to heat and light energy in a radiant heat lamp. A list of common kinds of energy with examples of the forms in which they are often manifest is given below:

Heat energy	Heat from the sun or a heat element.
Mechanical energy	Gravitational energy: an object having energy due to its height, say, a book on a shelf.
	Energy due to motion, say, a book falling from the shelf.
	Energy due to strain or distortion, say, the stretch of a spring.
Chemical energy	Energy stored in the chemical bonds of coal, petrol or glucose.
Electrical energy	Motion of charges, an electric current, magnetic attraction.

Radiation energy   Visible light, radio waves.

Energy of matter   Atomic fission, as in nuclear power generation.

Notice that, in the examples, what is being looked at is the conversion or transformation of one form of energy into another or into several others. In other words, energy is only evident during an energy change.

CONSERVATION OF ENERGY

It is important to understand that there is no beginning and no end to the processes of energy conversion. Energy can neither be created nor destroyed, only changed in form. The total amount of energy of a physical system always remains the same, no matter what energy conversions take place. This is the principle of the conservation of energy. Energy from nuclear power sources may seem to violate this principle in that energy is apparently created from nothing but, in fact, the energy is produced from that stored in the atomic structure of matter; a very small quantity of uranium is ultimately used up.

KINETIC AND POTENTIAL ENERGY

It can be seen that there are two general categories of energy. The one might be described as the energy of motion. It is called kinetic energy. The other is stored energy, referred to as potential energy. In the former, kinetic energy is seen in the movement of solid objects — the book falling from the shelf — or the motion of electric charges as an electric current. Examples of potential energy would be the position of the book on the shelf or the chemical bonding of glucose molecules, which release energy in the body when broken down. In some circumstances kinetic energy can be changed to potential energy and back again in a regular manner, forming an oscillating system. A swinging pendulum is an example of such a system in which the motion (kinetic energy) of the pendulum is converted to height (potential energy) at the extreme of each swing and back again. Similar mechanical oscillating systems are seen in many repetitive body motions such as walking.

MEASUREMENT OF ENERGY

Perhaps the simplest way to imagine energy is to consider the motion of a recognizable lump of matter. It has been noted above that if an object of 1 kg mass is given an acceleration of 1 m s^{-2} it experiences a force of 1 N. If such a force acts through a distance of 1 m it provides a *joule* of energy. So the unit of energy is the newton-metre or joule (J) (Table 1.1). In some contexts energy is referred to as *work* and so the unit of work is therefore also the joule. If a body possesses energy it has the ability to do work.

The joule is quite a small unit. Very approximately it is the amount of energy needed to lift this book 30 cm off a desk or the energy needed to stretch a 10 cm elastic band to three times its length. However, the joule describes the amount of energy and says nothing about the *rate of energy conversion*. In many situations it is this rate of energy change, the number of joules per second, that is of practical importance. Such a measure is called *power* and the units are called watts, so that:

$$1 \text{ watt} = 1 \text{ joule per second}$$

At other times and in other contexts energy has been described by a variety of units. It can be expressed in watts with the time specified, thus the watt-hour ($= 3600$ J) and the kilowatt-hour ($= 3.6 \times 10^6$ J). Other units of energy include the erg (10^{-7} J), which is used in some scientific contexts, the calorie (4.18 J) used in connection with heat energy and the Calorie (4.18×10^3 J) used in nutrition. This rather confusing situation of two units distinguished only by a capital letter has arisen for historical reasons; notice that:

$$1 \text{ Calorie} = 1 \text{ kilocalorie} = 1000 \text{ calories} = 4.18 \text{ kilojoules}$$

The further relationship of energy and matter is explained in Chapter 2.

2. *The structure of matter and materials*

All physical objects are formed of enormously diverse materials united in various complex ways. In order to understand why they have particular properties the huge variety of recognizable structures can be considered in terms of their constituent matter. Why, for example, can skin stretch? Why do dropped china cups break and why was animal tendon used in Roman catapults (ballistae)? In the study of biomechanics, it is important to understand not only the properties of human tissues but also those of the materials with which they interact.

Since there are many millions of substances, each one evidently different from the next, it is encouraging to be able to reduce this complexity. All are, in fact, made of combinations of about 90 naturally occurring substances called elements.

Table 2.1 Some elements occurring in the human body

Atomic number	Name	Symbol	Approximate relative atomic mass
1	Hydrogen	H	1
6	Carbon	C	12
7	Nitrogen	N	14
8	Oxygen	O	16
11	Sodium	Na	23
15	Phosphorus	P	31
16	Sulphur	S	32
17	Chlorine	Cl	35.5
19	Potassium	K	39
20	Calcium	Ca	40

ELEMENTS

Elements are made up of identical particles called *atoms*. There are, therefore, some 90 different kinds of atoms. Each of these elements and its constituent atoms is known by a chemical name and a recognized symbol. Table 2.1 lists some of the elements that are to hand, as it were! It will be noted that the symbols are simply the initial letters of the element, except for sodium and potassium, because sodium was originally called natrium and potassium kalium.

Apart from small quantities of many other elements – notably iron, magnesium, zinc, cobalt and copper – the human body is entirely made from the 10 elements in Table 2.1.

Thus when several of the same kinds of atoms are linked together the substance is called an element but if different kinds of atoms are united, a vast number of different substances are formed, called *compounds*. The unit due to the combining of two or more atoms is called a *molecule*. Molecules can be made of just two or several hundred atoms. Many of the molecules that make up living tissue are composed of long chains of repeating groups of a few atoms.

The basic building blocks of matter are therefore atoms. Understanding the nature of matter depends on understanding the atom.

ATOMS

Atoms are, of course, incredibly tiny. Even the largest could not possibly be seen directly (although there are techniques which enable the presence of atoms to be made evident in an indirect manner). The approximate diameter of an atom is 3×10^{-10} m, about 0.3 of a nanometre. To put it another way, if 100 million (10^8) atoms were lined up edge to edge they would form a line just about 3 cm long. The mass of each atom is commensurately small and hence rather inconvenient. The mass of the hydrogen atom is approximately 1.66×10^{-24} grams. Hydrogen is the simplest atom so it is easy to describe other atoms in terms of their relative mass, taking hydrogen as 1 unit. Nowadays, however, an isotope of carbon, carbon 12, is used as the accepted standard, its mass being equal to 12 times that of hydrogen. The mass of an atom is called the *atomic weight* of the atom for historical reasons but it is more sensible to call it the *relative atomic mass* (Table 2.1).

Atoms can be considered to be made up of still smaller discrete particles. The size of the atom was described above as being 3×10^{-10} m, but most of this is empty space. This, and much else, was elucidated in 1910 by the New Zealand scientist, Ernest Rutherford. He was able to deduce that most of the mass of the atom was found in a very small central region called the *nucleus*, which is associated with a positive charge. This nucleus has a diameter of about 10^{-14} m, so that the whole atom is some 10 000 times the size of the nucleus. (If the nucleus was scaled up to half a millimetre – like a pinhead – the atom would be the size of a large living room with a diameter of 5 m!) The space surrounding the nucleus is empty of particulate matter but is defined by negative charges moving at high speeds and called *electrons*. The simplest way to describe an atom is, therefore, a small, incredibly dense nucleus made up of particles, some of which have a positive charge, surrounded by electrons circling the nucleus at high speeds. This is often described as the planetary model because of its similarity to the planets orbiting the sun (Fig. 2.1). However, this is really too simple, because electrons can neither be thought of as little

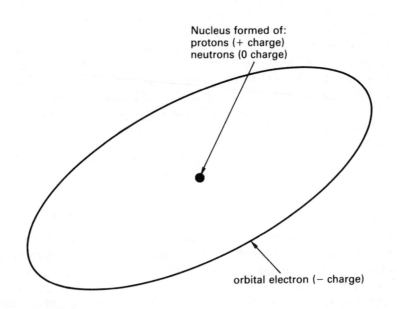

Nucleus formed of:
protons (+ charge)
neutrons (0 charge)

orbital electron (− charge)

Fig. 2.1 The planetary model of the atom.

particles — like tiny moving balls — nor as having clearly defined pathways around the nucleus. What can be described is the average position of electrons in relation to the nucleus — in other words the probability of finding an electron in that position (Fig. 2.2). This pathway, called an *orbital* or *shell*, is often, but not always, spherical around the central nucleus. When one electron is circling the nucleus, as occurs in a hydrogen atom, it is easy to imagine its average motion in the plane of the shell of an egg, with the yolk as the nucleus. Each orbital has a definite capacity for electrons, after which it is full. Two electrons can circle in the first orbital or shell, as occurs in the helium atom. However, if the atom has more than two electrons these move in spherical shells outside the first. In fact an atom is composed of a nucleus with electrons circling in a series of concentric shells, each a greater average distance from the nucleus and containing electrons which have a specific pattern of movement different from every other electron.

The nucleus contains two kinds of particles, *protons* which have a positive charge and *neutrons* which have no charge. Both of these have significant and similar masses. They are said to have a mass number of 1. The positive charge of the proton exactly balances the negative charge of the electron so that, as atoms are electrically neutral, the number of electrons in its orbital must be the same as the number of protons in its nucleus. Thus in the hydrogen atom there is one proton in the nucleus and one electron in an orbital. Similarly, the helium atom contains two

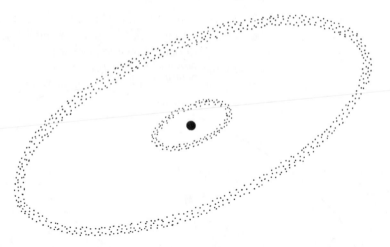

Fig. 2.2 The uncertainty model of the atom. Representation of the spatial probability distribution for electrons in their first two principal quantum numbers.

electrons and two protons. Atoms of different elements contain characteristic numbers of protons and electrons for that atom and hence that element. The number of protons (and hence electrons) is given by the *atomic number* (Z) (Table 2.1). The number of protons plus neutrons is given by the mass number (the whole number closest to the relative atomic mass).

If the relative atomic masses are compared with the atomic numbers in Table 2.1 it will be noticed that all the elements except hydrogen are twice, or a little more than twice, the mass of their atomic number. This means that the other particles in the nuclei, the neutrons, contribute to the mass and are at least as numerous as the protons. In fact most atoms, especially the heavier atoms, contain more neutrons than protons.

As noted earlier, elements are made up of atoms that are chemically identical to one another. However, they do not necessarily have exactly the same relative atomic masses. The difference is accounted for by atoms that contain different numbers of neutrons. They are called *isotopes*. If an element has different isotopes, the relative atomic mass is not a whole number but reflects the average; see chlorine in Table 2.1. In fact Table 2.1 shows whole numbers for simplicity but many elements are mixtures with very small numbers of isotopes. For instance the relative atomic mass of carbon (C) is strictly 12.01115 because of small quantities of ^{13}C and ^{14}C; however, nearly 99% consists of ^{12}C.

In summary, a simple model of the atom can be described as consisting of a central nucleus containing the mass of the atom and composed of positively charged protons and unchanged neutrons surrounded by a relatively large space in which rapidly moving, negatively charged electrons circulate. This is further summarized in Table 2.2.

In a neutral atom the number of protons is equal to the number of electrons. However, if one or more electrons are removed, the particle becomes positively charged and is no longer called an atom. Similarly, if one or more electrons are added it becomes negatively charged. In both cases the atom with a deficiency or excess of electrons is called an *ion* (derived from a Greek word meaning going, in the sense of wandering, since ions in fluids are able to move about).

Table 2.2 Particles of an atom

Particle	Charge	Mass number
Proton	+	1
Neutron	0	1
Electron	−	0

QUANTUM NUMBERS

What has been noted so far is very simplistic. As already mentioned, atoms consist of a number of shells or orbitals numbered from that nearest to the nucleus, called 1, outwards. The shell number is given by the *principal quantum number* (n). The electron shells are made up of one or more subshells which represent different energy levels. These subshells are described by the *second quantum number* (l) and are numbered from 0 upwards. Each subshell can contain a limited number of electrons. These are specified by letters, thus: s can hold 2 electrons, p can hold 6, d 10 and f 14. In a magnetic field these subshells can be further subdivided into orbitals which each hold up to two electrons. This is given by the third or magnetic quantum number (m). The two electrons found in the same orbital turn out to be spinning in opposite directions. This spin is independent of the motion of the electron around the nucleus but is motion of the electron on its own axis. The direction of spin is indicated by the fourth or spin quantum number (s) and can only be one of two possibilities, thought of as either clockwise or anticlockwise. Thus the distribution of electrons in an element, its electronic configuration, and the energy of each electron is different from that of every other electron in the atom (the Pauli exclusion principle) and can be described in terms of the four quantum numbers.

An analogy for the atom is the Roman amphitheatre. The nucleus is the central stage and the electrons are the individual people in the audience. Seats have to be filled from the bottom, nearest the stage, first. The principal quantum numbers (n) represent banks of seats. The subshells (l) are individual rows of seats. The third quantum number (m) is a pair of seats and the fourth (s), rather fancifully, is the way each individual faces (Fig. 2.3).

The lowest possible energy level is the *ground state*: n = 1. The

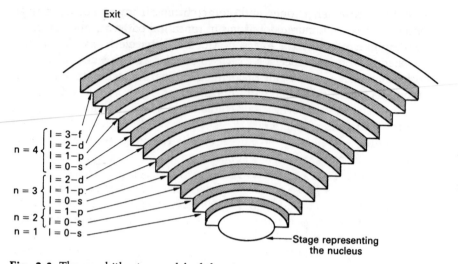

Exit

$n = 4$ $\begin{cases} l = 3-f \\ l = 2-d \\ l = 1-p \\ l = 0-s \end{cases}$

$n = 3$ $\begin{cases} l = 2-d \\ l = 1-p \\ l = 0-s \end{cases}$

$n = 2$ $\begin{cases} l = 1-p \\ l = 0-s \end{cases}$

$n = 1$ $\quad l = 0-s$

Stage representing the nucleus

Fig. 2.3 The amphitheatre model of the atom.

minimum energy required to remove an electron from an atom in its ground state is the *ionization energy*. The energy required to remove successive electrons increases. The most easily removed electron is held with the smallest force because it is furthest from the nucleus. The most tightly bound is closest to the nucleus and has a high ionization energy. When atoms interact with one another it is the outermost electrons that will be involved. In fact, the amount of energy holding the outermost electron determines its chemical reactivity; in other words, the way in which the atom will react with other atoms to form molecules. It is called the *first ionization energy* and varies from atom to atom. It is, of course, a measure of how tightly the outer electron is held to the nucleus. In the same way electronic configuration is linked to chemical behaviour and accounts for the grouping of elements into families in the periodic table. The elements that have a full outer shell of electrons and high first ionization energies tend to be inert. Those that readily lose or gain an electron are especially reactive and have low first ionization energies.

Returning to the amphitheatre analogy − if the exits are only at the top of the theatre, ionization energy is the minimum energy required for a person to reach the exit and first ionization energy is the energy required by the person in the highest occupied level of seats. Thus the nearer the stage (the nucleus) the person (electron) is sitting, the more energy is needed to reach the exit.

As mentioned earlier, atoms from different elements join to form compounds; molecules are the smallest possible amount of an element or compound. The formation of the millions of possible molecules, some simply pairs of identical atoms (e.g. H_2), others sheets or chains of different atoms connected together, depends on the union of one atom to another. Some of those, notably the biological molecules, are made almost entirely of carbon, hydrogen and oxygen atoms. They can be quite large, being made up of hundreds of atoms in repeating patterns. This linking or bonding is effected by the interaction of the outer electrons. One way is the sharing of pairs of electrons, *covalent bonding* as it is called. This forms molecules made up of a pair of identical atoms. An opposite way is the union of atoms with different ionization energies. Thus sodium and chlorine can unite to form a salt (sodium chloride). Sodium has a single electron in its outer shell which is easily removed, rendering it a positive ion. Chlorine, on the other hand, lacks an electron to complete its outer shell. If it gains an electron it will become a negative ion. The sodium ion and the chlorine ion will attract each other, the opposite charges serving to hold the atoms into a molecule. This is called *ionic bonding* and in this instance forms crystals of sodium chloride. What is happening in the formation of molecules is rather like the building of very large atoms with several nuclei and shared electrons.

The sharing of electrons in many molecules is not always equal, which causes a charge to exist between the two ends of the molecule, one end being positive relative to the other. This is called a *dipole*. Such polar molecules, the water molecule for example, are readily influenced by an electric field due to their charge.

Changes that are recognized as chemical reactions, such as an explosion, the rusting of iron or the digestion of food, are all rearrangements of atoms at a molecular level in which some bonds are ruptured and new ones are fashioned. In some circumstances, such as the explosion, energy is released. This is the more obvious because the chemical reaction is very rapid. A similar release of mechanical energy may be brought about by changes in chemical bonding during the contraction of a muscle but the rate of energy release occurs more slowly.

From what has been described so far it might be concluded that the protons, neutrons and electrons are fundamental particles, that is, they are not made up of smaller subunits. This may well be a reasonable assertion as far as the electron is concerned, but not for the others. Furthermore, at this subatomic level it becomes impossible to think of particles in terms of solid objects; their energy must be taken into account.

The atom can only have certain definite amounts of energy represented by the quantum numbers. However, the electron can jump between these levels. If an electron changes its orbital to one nearer the nucleus with a lower energy level, energy is released from the atom in the form of a packet or unit of electromagnetic radiation called a *photon*. The frequency and energy of this radiation depend on the energy released by the electron. The photon, however, travels away from the atom and can react with other atoms. It is effectively an energy particle.

By giving the nucleus of the atom a great deal of energy — by colliding protons and neutrons with one another — various other particles have been found. One would expect that protons, having like charges, would repel each other but, in general, protons and neutrons are held together firmly in the atomic nucleus. The force uniting them is called the *strong force.* The particles discovered during these collisions together with the particles called *pions* are collectively called *hadrons* (derived from a Greek word meaning bulky because they are relatively large particles). Other particles are formed during interactions in the nucleus. These include the electron and a similar but positively charged particle called a *positron,* as well as an uncharged particle called a *neutrino* and other particles called *muons.* These are collectively labelled *leptons.* Table 2.3 summarizes various particles.

Table 2.3 Hadrons, leptons and the photon

Hadrons		Leptons		The photon
Proton	+	Positron	+	A packet of electromagnetic energy
Pion	+			
	−	Electron	−	
	0			
Neutron	0	Neutrino	0	
		Muon	+	
			−	

None of this invalidates the model of the atom based on protons, neutrons and electrons but it indicates that the interaction of energy and matter is the basis of structure at a subatomic level. In fact, the laws of conservation of energy become merged at this level and can be represented by the well known equation

$$E = mc^2$$

(energy = mass × velocity of electromagnetic radiation squared)

Thus an increase in mass is always associated with a decrease in energy and an increase in energy with a decrease in mass. This is what happens in the sun or in the nuclear reactor of a power station where nuclear fission converts small amounts of matter into large amounts of energy.

STATES OF MATTER

So far the nature of the microstructure of matter has been considered in terms of atoms and molecules but the characteristics of matter depend on the way these atoms and molecules are held together. Under the temperature and pressure conditions that exist at the surface of the earth,

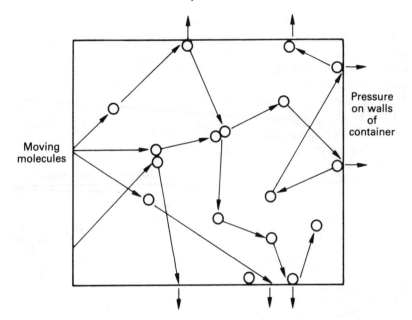

Fig. 2.4 Zigzag pathways of molecules – Brownian motion.

matter can exist as gases, liquids or solids. (In fact, there are some substances that do not fit exactly into one of these categories.) Further, alterations of the temperature and/or pressure can effect a change of state. It is helpful to consider the three states of matter separately.

GASES

Gases are the most diffuse form of matter, a form in which there is least structure and in which the atoms or molecules are widely separated from one another. The wide separations allow rapid and random movement of the molecules or atoms. This movement, which can be made visible with a microscope under suitable conditions, is called *Brownian motion* (after the Scottish botanist, Robert Brown, 1773–1858). It consists of irregular zigzag motion as each particle collides with others and bounces off again. Particles will also strike the sides of a container holding the gas. These collisions are elastic so that energy may be transferred from molecule to molecule but is not lost. In fact, this energy of motion – kinetic energy – is part of the energy held in the microstructure of all matter which is recognized as heat. Typical pathways are shown diagrammatically in Figure 2.4. This *kinetic theory* of gases, as it is called, can be summarized by the following points:

1. The distances between the molecules or atoms are enormous compared with the size of the particle itself.

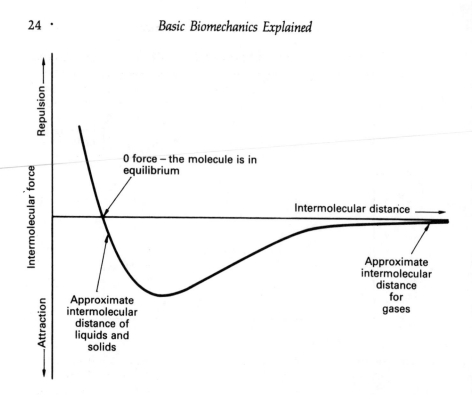

Fig. 2.5 Representation of forces related to intermolecular distance.

2. The molecules are in constant, rapid, random, straight-line motion.
3. Because of the distances between them, intermolecular forces are neglible except during collisions.

These account for the well known characteristics of gases, notably the *universal gas law* which describes the interrelationship of the volume, pressure and temperature for any given sample of gas:

$$\frac{PV}{T} = \text{number of moles of gas} \times \text{the universal gas constant (R)}^*$$

where P = pressure, V = volume and T = temperature.

This is combining Boyle's law, the pressure–volume relationship and Charles's law, the volume–temperature relationship. Thus if temperature is constant the pressure of a given volume of gas is inversely proportional to its volume and if pressure is constant the volume of the gas varies with temperature. The pressure is due to the collisions of molecules with the walls of the container. Decreasing the volume, i.e. pushing the molecules closer together, and increasing the amount of movement by heating will both increase the number of collisions on the walls, thus increasing the

*Gas constant R = 8.314 J K^{-1} mol^{-1}

pressure. Similarly, gases can expand to fill an available volume because the molecules can move further apart. The constant irregular motion also accounts for diffusion which occurs when two gases mix at a rate which depends on their temperature. The universal gas law is not exactly true for gases at very high pressure (at which the volume of the gas molecules themselves becomes significant) and for gases at very low temperature (when the attractive forces between molecules – van der Waals forces, as they are called – slow the molecular motion).

As well as forces of attraction between atoms and molecules there must be repulsive forces or they would collapse. The force of attraction between oppositely charged ions is balanced by the electron clouds repelling each other. In a solid the molecules must be more or less in equilibrium. If solids are compressed the forces of repulsion increase and if stretched the forces of attraction increase. A graph of force related to intermolecular distance is represented in Figure 2.5. There is zero force when the molecules are in equilibrium.

In gases the average distance between centres of molecules or atoms is quite large when compared with that of solids and liquids. For a gas at $0°C$ and 1 atmosphere pressure the average intermolecular distance is about 3.3 nanometres (3.3×10^{-9} m). In liquids and solids the average distance is about a tenth of this. This distance is very close to the point at which the electron clouds of adjacent molecules intermingle sufficiently to produce repulsion forces between molecules (Fig. 2.5).

LIQUIDS

Liquids have a definite volume and density, unlike gases, and take the shape of any container influenced by gravity. They are not rigid but are hard to compress. The density of a liquid is very much the same as that of the equivalent solid but very much greater than that of the gas. Thus a drop of water increases in volume some 1600 times when it is converted to water vapour, i.e. a gas. As noted above, the molecules of liquid are very close together so that the volume of liquid is very much less affected by pressure and temperature changes than that of gas. Due to the closeness of molecules in liquids the average distance moved during random motion is much less than that of gases. The average distance travelled by a molecule between collisions, called the mean free path, is perhaps tens of nanometres in a gas but only tiny fractions of a nanometre in liquids.

While the density of liquids and close proximity of their molecules make them very like solids, the free random movement of their molecules, albeit over short distances, makes them behave like gases. That is to say, Brownian movement can be observed; they flow and those with similar molecules will diffuse with one another. However, in some instances it is very difficult to make two liquids mix together – oil and water, for example – a fact that is of considerable biological importance. It is also well recognized that liquids differ greatly from one another in the ease with which they flow – a property called viscosity. This is simply a function of how easily the molecules will move in respect to one another and is unrelated to density. Water and alcohol are well known liquids of low viscosity, while blood, treacle and thick oil have high viscosity. Unsurprisingly, viscosity falls with increasing temperature since this brings about more molecular movement.

SOLIDS

Solids are clearly different from liquids and gases, which together are known as fluids, because of their rigidity of structure – they do not conform to the shape of their container. They are usually classified into crystalline and amorphous solids. Amorphous solids, such as certain plastics or glass, are in some ways on the boundary between liquids and solids, whereas crystalline solids are formed of regular, repeating arrays of atoms in a three-dimensional structure. The basic unit cell of such structures consists of a number of atoms or molecules in a more or less fixed relationship. There are seven different geometric arrangements to form the unit cell: cubic (like sodium chloride), tetragonal, orthorhombic, rhombohedral, monoclinic, triclinic and hexagonal. These arrays of crystals, called a crystal lattice, are held together by different forces in different substances. Thus:

1. Atoms held together by van der Waals forces or dipole interactions are called *molecular solids*. Their relatively weak, intermolecular forces mean that they melt easily and form soft crystals. Sulphur and solid carbon dioxide (dry ice) are examples. Other molecular solids are linked by hydrogen bonding. These form rather stronger bonds, forming harder crystals, ice being the most important example.
2. *Covalent bonding* links the atoms in the crystals together in a strong bond with fixed angles between atoms forming very hard, high-melting-point crystals, such as diamonds and quartz. This is rather like fixing the atoms in the crystals into a sort of supermolecule. The atoms share their electrons.
3. *Ionic bonds* are formed when strong electrostatic forces hold the oppositely charged ions together. This is the bonding form of sodium chloride.
4. *Metallic solids* are like a mass of metal ions with positive charges in a sea of electrons. The electrons wander freely through the crystal lattice rather than belonging to a single atom. This accounts for the electrical and thermal conductivity of metals. Of course in an uncharged piece of metal the total number of electrons is equal to the total number of protons. In many metals there is also some covalent bonding, which accounts for the variations of melting points and qualities such as hardness or brittleness of different metals.

This special crystalline structure of metals accounts for other properties. The crystal lattice of positive ions in a negatively charged 'fluid' means that abrupt stress, such as a blow with a hammer, can force the ions together. These then reform the original lattice structure when the compression ceases because of the repulsion forces between ions and attraction to the surrounding electrons. This gives metals their elastic properties. Further, because the crystal lattice arrangement is regular and uniform, planes of ions can slide over one another by a few lattice spacings and yet retain their symmetry. This accounts for the way in which most metals can be worked, e.g. hammered flat or drawn out into wires, when they are said to be ductile.

In spite of the bonding considered above it would be a mistake to think of atoms and molecules in solids as being stationary. They are in constant vibratory motion which, of course, increases with rising temperature.

Crystal lattices are not pure and structurally perfect. Real solids often have deficiencies in the crystal lattice, called lattice vacancies, and sometimes the lattice is irregular − lattice dislocations.

HOW SOLIDS SUPPORT LOADS

A solid is described, indeed defined, as rigid. This means that the material of which it is made is able to resist a mechanical force. The fact that it remains solid means that it is able to sustain its own weight, i.e. resist the force of gravity. It is the old question of why the table is able to support the book, the chair support the reader, the floor support the table and the chair, and so on. The answer is that when an object presses on another − like the book on the table − the second object presses back with equal force, i.e. the table presses back on the book.

It will be recalled that Newton's first and second laws of motion were considered in Chapter 1. What has just been described is enshrined in Newton's third law: if a body A exerts a force on body B, then body B exerts an equal but opposite force on body A. This is sometimes expressed as: every action has an equal and opposite reaction.

This suits the example used above, but implies, erroneously, that the second force occurs after the first. This applies not only to objects pressing against other objects but equally to those that are pulling apart: the famous apple hanging from a tree (and eventually falling, for Newton's alleged moment of insight!). It is easy to understand the one force exerted by body A, e.g. the pressure of the feet on the floor due to the weight of the owner of the feet, or the pulling down on a strap fixed in the roof of a train, but perhaps not as easy to recognize how a passive object, like the floor or the roof, can provide the opposite force. In the words of the thoughtful 12-year-old on having Newton's third law explained, 'If the floor is pushing up while I am standing on it why doesn't it come up when I step away?' The answer is that it does. This, however, is not obvious except on such surfaces as springboards or 'bouncy castles'. What enables the other object — object B — to push or pull back is the fact that after it is distorted it returns to its original shape, i.e. it is *elastic*. This quality of elasticity is central to the way in which matter, materials and structures interact. In fact, every structure must deform to some extent when a force or load is applied to it. Thus, at each footstep not only is the articular cartilage of the knee and hip compressed a little but the apparently rigid tibia and femur are bent to a very small degree. Elasticity is concerned with the interaction between the forces, or *stress*, and the deformation, or *strain*, in matter and structures. This concept is associated with the English scientist, Robert Hooke, who formulated what became known as Hooke's law. In 1679 Hooke published a paper containing the statement, 'Ut tensio sic vis' (as the extension so the force). What he wrote was:

The power of any Spring is in the same proportion with the Tension [meaning extension] thereof: that is, if one power stretch or bend it one space, two will bend it two, three will bend it three and so forward. And this is the Rule or Law of Nature upon which all manner of Restituent or Springing motion doth proceed.

A modern, more succinct version is usually given as 'strain is proportional to the stress producing it'. The centrally important concept is that distortion is proportional to the force producing it. It is the atoms and molecules of which the material is made that behave in this elastic manner. Hence the bulk of the material, and any structure that it forms, behaves in the same way. Thus the forces of attraction and repulsion between atoms and molecules are involved so that when a material is compressed the average intermolecular distance is decreased (see Fig. 2.5), and thus the force of repulsion is increased. Similarly, stretching causes an increase in the force of attraction. Elasticity is easily associated with materials that stretch and recover readily, such as rubber bands, but less obviously with more rigid materials such as stone and bone. The difference is in the *stiffness*, that is it takes more force to deform stone than rubber. No material can be absolutely rigid but hard gem stones like diamonds are extremely stiff.

The word stress was used loosely above to describe the applied force but what matters is the force applied per unit area. Thus:

$$\text{stress} = \frac{\text{force}}{\text{area}}$$

Stress can be quoted in any units of force per unit area but the appropriate SI units are newtons per square metre, hence $N\,m^{-2}$. One newton per square metre is 1 pascal. Pascals are known as units of pressure. Stress within a solid is the same as pressure in a fluid. Other units of stress or pressure are often encountered, e.g. psi (pounds per square inch). Large stresses are measured in meganewtons per square metre

(MN m^{-2}). It should be emphasized that pressure or stress in a material acts at a point and is not necessarily spread over any particular area, although its magnitude must be described in this way. Also, the word stress has this very specific meaning, in this context, and should not be confused with its use to describe psychological or physiological states.

The word strain is used to describe the distortion − change of shape − that occurs in a solid due to an applied stress. As it is describing a change, it is expressed as the ratio of the original shape to that after the force has been applied. For example, the strain in a piece of elastic being stretched is:

$$\frac{\text{the increased length}}{\text{the original length}}$$

As strain is a ratio, it has no units, it is just a number. Thus strain describes how far the molecules of a solid are being pulled apart or pushed together while stress describes the force with which this happens (see Fig. 2.5).

When comparing similar sized pieces of different materials, the *stiffness*, as opposed to the *flexibility*, is readily recognized. Thus a rubber band stretches easily while a piece of string does not. What is being recognized is the relationship between the force or stress used and the resulting stretch or strain. This can be expressed more precisely by plotting a graph of stress against strain. The stress–strain diagram is characteristic of any given material and, within limits, will be a straight line whose slope, or gradient, describes the stiffness of the material. The steeper the gradient, the stiffer the material. Thus the ratio of stress to strain is a constant known as *Young's modulus*, denoted E. The idea is illustrated by the different slopes of the stress–strain diagram shown in Figure 2.6 for various materials. Young's modulus for any material can thus be given as a figure, which is the stress, in N m^{-2}, divided by the strain. Since strain is a ratio with no units, Young's modulus is given in N m^{-2}. Table 2.4 gives examples of Young's modulus for some familiar materials and human tissues. It must be noted that the tissues and some other materials shown are not uniform compounds or elements. It can be seen that these materials become increasingly stiff or less flexible the further their position down the list.

PLASTICITY

It will have been noted that elastic properties were described above with the proviso 'within certain limits' and that Figure 2.6 shows that distortion cannot occur indefinitely with increasing stress. What happens, in most materials, is a rapidly increasing distortion once the stress goes beyond a certain point referred to as its *elastic limit*. Beyond this, *plastic deformation* occurs and is characterized by the fact that, when the stress is released, the

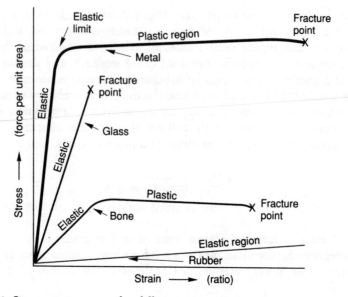

Fig. 2.6 Stress–strain curves for different materials.

Table 2.4 Young's modulus of various materials

Substance	Young's modulus (MN m^{-2})
Rubber	7
Cartilage	24
Tendon	600
Plastics, e.g. polythene/nylon	1 400
Plywood	7 000
Bone	21 000
Glass	70 000
Iron/steel	210 000
Diamond	1 200 000

Data from Gordon, 1978.

material does not recover its original shape, but it remains distorted. This was noted above as the ductile property of metals. The mechanism of plastic deformation is not the same in every material. In metals it is due to slip between parts of the crystal lattice arrangement. This generally occurs at sites where the lattice is defective, called dislocations. Other materials, such as plastic polymers, suffer permanent distortion as their long chain molecules realign in the direction of the stress.

FRACTURE

Continuing the applied stress through plastic deformation ultimately causes the material to break, with complete separation of the molecules from one another. This is called the failure point, or fracture point, or, if tension is being tested, the ultimate tensile strength. Some materials deform plastically a great deal before final fracture, while others, such as glass, break without plastic deformation. Such materials are called *brittle*. These ideas are shown on the stress–strain graphs in Figure 2.6. The higher the fracture point, the stronger the material.

The stress point at which the material breaks can be described in $MN\,m^{-2}$, but it should be understood that this, as well as Young's modulus, depends on the type of stress applied. Examples of the tensile strength of various materials are given in Table 2.5. It will be seen that metals appear to have higher values, but it must be realized that they have much higher density than, say, plant or animal tissues, so that for an equivalent weight they are not necessarily stronger.

Table 2.5 Tensile strength of various materials

Material	Tensile strength ($MN\,m^{-2}$)
Cartilage	3
Skin	10.3
Tendon	82
Hemp rope	82
Bone	110
Hair	192
Spider's web	240
Catgut	350
Mild steel	400
Nylon thread	1050
High tensile engineering steel	1550

Modified from Gordon, 1978.

Young's modulus has been considered in respect of direct stress – tension or compression – but the same relationship exists between shear stress and shear strain, which may be called the modulus of rigidity and denoted G. Shear loading occurs when stress is applied in opposite directions on the two sides of the material, causing it to deform internally in an angular manner (see Fig. 2.7). A third elastic modulus is called the bulk modulus, K, where the stress is equal over the whole surface and the strain is the change in volume of the material. The elastic moduli of

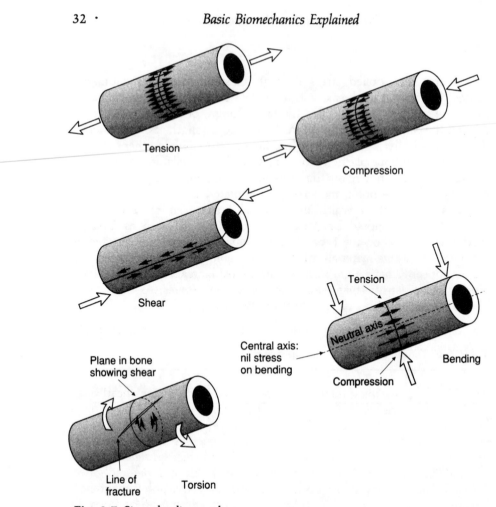

Fig. 2.7 Stress loading on bone.

materials are often different for tension, compression, shear etc. and in most situations forces applied to human or animal tissues are complex, with several different forces being applied at once.

The stress–strain plots of Figure 2.6 are representations of force and distance and, as noted in Chapter 1, energy is force multiplied by distance; 1 N acting through 1 m gives 1 J of energy. The area under the stress–strain graph is therefore proportional to the stored energy. Thus, in the elastic region the amount of energy that can be returned on elastic recovery can be measured, as can the energy absorbed in the material under the plastic region. The area under the elastic part of the stress–strain plot is the strain energy and is: stress × strain × 1/2. These ideas are illustrated for a hypothetical material in Figure 2.8. As will be considered later, the ability of tissues to store and return energy is of enormous importance for all kinds of human and animal activities. Elasticity of tissues is essential for making human walking, or kangaroo bounding, so efficient

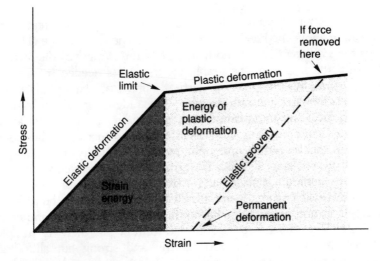

Fig. 2.8 Stress–strain graph of hypothetical material to illustrate plastic deformation and energy storage.

or indeed for smoothing the force of the ejected blood at each heart beat. The amount of energy that can be stored in a given volume or given mass of the tissue or material is the important feature. The energy that can be stored in joules per kilogram for some familiar materials is shown in Table 2.6. Bronze is often used to make hairsprings, and steel springs are found in many situations, such as car suspensions or to close doors and gates. The well known English longbows were made of yew wood (though not, apparently, English yew). It is striking how much energy can be stored in tendon, hence its use in Roman ballistae, and even more in rubber.

The energy applied to effect plastic deformation remains in the microstructure of the material and some appears as heat. Bending a piece of malleable metal rapidly to and fro by hand in order to break it leads to quite marked heating, which can sometimes be felt quite easily.

Table 2.6 Maximum strain energy stored

Material	Stored energy body ($J\,kg^{-1}$)
Bronze	70
Spring steel	130
Yew wood	900
Tendon	2500
Rubber	8000

SUMMARY

The stress–strain plots of Figures 2.6 and 2.8 give a great deal of information about the behaviour of materials. The slope of the elastic part shows the *stiffness* (Young's modulus), while the *strength* of the material is shown by the height of the graph, i.e. the stress needed to break it in $N m^{-2}$. Further, the *energy stored* elastically and that *absorbed* plastically is indicated in the area beneath the plot. These ideas can be illustrated in a simple practical, but unmeasured, way by bending the plastic of an (old!) credit card. Gentle bending allows elastic recoil to occur. Further bending causes deformation which does not recover elastically and still greater force leads to breaking. It is also interesting and instructive to consider the features of common objects and materials in terms of their relative stiffness (elasticity), strength and plastic deformation. Thus the toothbrush is stiff and strong while the metal toothpaste tube is flexible and deforms plastically. The china cup is stiff and brittle, i.e. there is no plastic deformation. The metal teaspoon is stiff and strong but allows great plastic deformation with sufficient force. The biscuit is weak unless dunked when it becomes more flexible!

MECHANICAL PROPERTIES OF THE TISSUES

The dominant mechanical features of bone are stiffness and strength, as discussed below. Cartilage, while having similar strength, is much more flexible. This is particularly true of elastic cartilage such as that found in the external ear. The collagenous tissues, ligaments and tendons, are strong, flexible and elastic. The actual properties of all collagenous tissues depend on the nature of the fibres, their properties and orientation. Skin is very evidently flexible and elastic, this being largely due to the arrangement of collagen fibres and the presence of elastic fibres in the dermis. Tissues and organs that regularly need to adjust their size to accommodate different volumes and pressures, such as the aorta, stomach, bladder and uterus, are made appropriately strong and elastic. Thus, the aorta is extremely strong to be able to resist rupture by the high systolic pressure exerted during ventricular systole and is highly elastic. Large veins, on the other hand, are flexible and elastic but much weaker, since they are subjected to negligible pressures. Some of these tissues are considered in more detail below.

BONE

Bone is a composite tissue formed of strong collagenous fibres enmeshing a hard mineral crystalline material, calcium apatite. It also contains blood vessels, fat and nerves. Individual bones and parts of bones are made of different amounts of mineralized bone; the *porosity*, expressed as a percentage, is the proportion of the bone's volume occupied by non-mineralized tissue. A simple distinction is usually made between cortical or dense bone, found on the bone surface and especially in the shafts of long bones, and cancellous bone, found in the body of most bones and expanded ends of long bones. The former have porosities of between 5% and 30%, while the latter have porosities of 30% to 90%. Clearly, the distinction between the two types is arbitrary. Cortical bone is stiffer than cancellous but the latter will store more energy before fracture. Young's modulus for cancellous bone is typically about a fifth of that of cortical bone. (A range of 7000–21 000 MN m^{-2} for cortical and 700–4900 MN m^{-2} for cancellous bone is given for Young's modulus (Radin *et al.* 1992).)

Stress loading on bone

Forces can be applied as tension, compression, shear or combined loading, such as bending or torsion. Behaviour of the bone is somewhat different in each of the stress modes.

In *tension*, equal and opposite forces pull away from the bone (see Fig. 2.7). The maximum stress will be in a plane perpendicular to the direction of the applied forces inside the bone. The stretched part of the bone will narrow a very small amount and, if the force is increased to fracture point, the osteons (minute cylindrical units of bone tissue) pull apart. Such fractures are recognized clinically as avulsion fractures: of the calcaneus due to contraction of triceps surae; of the patella or tibial tubercle due to contraction of quadriceps; or of the medial malleolus in some fracture-dislocations of the ankle, for example.

In *compression*, equal and opposite forces are applied to the bone, the maximum stress also being in a plane perpendicular to the applied load (see Fig. 2.7). The affected part of the bone shortens and widens and ultimately a fracture occurs with oblique cracking of the osteons. Compression fractures are recognized clinically as crush fractures, e.g. calcaneus, vertebrae or impacted fractures such as Colles, surgical neck of the humerus or transtrochanteric in the upper end of the femur.

In *shear* stress, the force is applied parallel to the surface of the bone, the stress being maximum in a plane parallel to the applied forces. This will cause angular distortion within the bone (see Fig. 2.7). Clinically, shear forces cause such injuries as vertical fractures in the tibial plateau or chip fractures of the head of the radius.

Bending is due to forces acting to cause the bone to distort about a neutral axis. It involves compression on one side and tension on the other side of the bone but no stress in the very centre at the neutral axis (see Fig. 2.7). The size of the stress in the bone is proportional to its distance from the neutral axis and is greatest at the surface. Since material at the centre of a rod, therefore, contributes nothing to its ability to resist bending, it is sensible to make structures such as bicycle frames or walking frames from metal tubing. Similarly, the shafts of long bones are hollow, but bone is more triangular than circular in cross-section so that the compression and tension stresses are not necessarily equal. Bending may lead to fracture due to the two ends of a bone being fixed while a third force is applied between the ends under which the fracture occurs, as in Figure 2.7. This occurs where a blow near the centre of a long bone causes a fracture, such as a fractured mid-shaft of the ulna. Alternatively, the two ends of the bone can be moved relative to one another to cause a fracture at some point (the weakest point) in the shaft. This occurs in a fracture of the clavicle due to a fall on the arm.

Torsion means twisting about an axis and causes shear stress throughout the bone which, like bending, is greater further from the central axis (see Fig. 2.7). As well as shear stress, torsion causes tension and compression in planes diagonal to the axis. This is why bone loaded in torsion tends to fracture in an oblique or spiral line. The effect can be demonstrated by firmly twisting a rod of any easily broken solid; a blackboard chalk is often used. Spiral or oblique fractures, such as of the tibial shaft, are invariably due to torsion such as rotating the upper end of the tibia about a fixed foot or ankle.

What has just been described provides some insight into the mechanisms of clinical fractures but it must be realized that many real life situations are much more complex. The stress acts in several modes at once and living bone is highly irregular in shape. Consequently the precise prediction of the results of applying particular forces becomes impossible. This is further complicated by the fact that both the stiffness and the ultimate stress (strength) for a particular mode of applied force varies with its orientation in the bone. Thus the stress–strain graph for tension in the femur is much more vertical (stiffer) and reaches a higher ultimate stress (stronger) if applied in the long axis of the femur, as illustrated in Figure 2.7. If applied at an angle or transversely across the bone it is less stiff and weaker (Frankel and Burstein, 1970).

Bone strength

One very important feature of bone tissue is that, being a mixture of materials, it exhibits different properties with different modes of stress. Thus cortical bone is very much stronger, i.e. it has higher ultimate stress in compression than in shear, and somewhat higher than in tension (Reilly and Burstein, 1975). This is due to the fact that tension and compression are resisted by the collagen fibres and mineral content respectively. Bone is a composite material, like reinforced concrete, which is naturally strong in compression but needs the embedded steel rods to enable it to resist tension forces. In many buildings prestressed concrete is used, in which the steel rods are stretched before the concrete sets so that, when it is set, the rods try to recover their initial length, causing compression of the concrete. This makes the concrete beam stronger since it is in

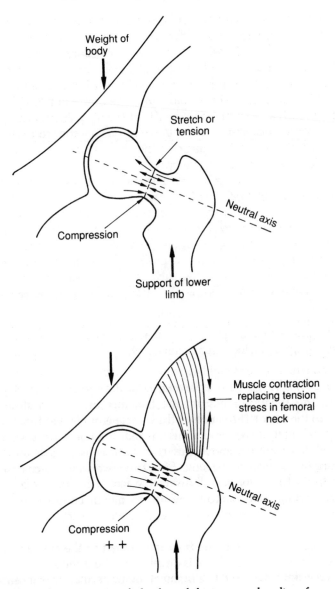

Weight of body

Stretch or tension

Neutral axis

Compression

Support of lower limb

Muscle contraction replacing tension stress in femoral neck

Neutral axis

Compression
+ +

Fig. 2.9 Effect of contraction of the hip abductors on bending force in the femoral neck.

compression. Thus the side in tension, when it is bent, has to be decompressed before it can be stretched in tension to ultimate fracture. The principle of prestressing is used in the body by recruiting muscle contraction to decrease tensile stresses on the bone. There are many examples of muscle contracting on the tension side of long bones subjected to bending. Figure 2.9 illustrates the effect of contraction of the short hip abductors, gluteus medius and minimus, to reduce tension in the

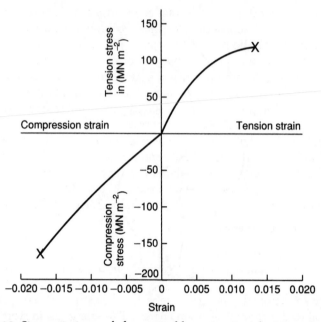

Fig. 2.10 Stress–strain graph for cortical bone (see text for Young's moduli and ultimate strengths; modified from Cromer, 1981).

upper and outer part of the femoral neck during weightbearing. (Other forces fixing the femur ensure that bending rather than shear force is applied to the neck.) The action of the muscle ensures that tension stress in the superior part of the femoral neck is reduced but compression stress is increased. It was noted above that cortical bone is considerably stronger in compression than in tension. Similar prestressing mechanisms occur elsewhere in the body and illustrate the fact that bones are not simply rigid supporting members to be moved by muscle contraction, but part of a complex dynamic body structure constantly reacting to the applied loads.

The structure of bone tissue is clearly related to the applied stresses, so that dense strong cortical bone is developed where the stress is greatest. It is also considered that the alignment of trabeculae in cancellous bone reflects the pattern of stress habitually applied. This is evident in a coronal section through the femoral neck in which the dense cortical bone to resist compression is seen on the inferior part of the neck (see Fig. 2.9). However, it is very difficult to make exact predictions or correlations of bone structure to its functions, because of the extreme complexity of the matter. This also applies to the physical parameters considered above, Young's modulus, ultimate stress etc., so that where figures are given these should be considered as representative rather than exact. Nevertheless, Figure 2.10 shows the behaviour of cortical bone under both tension and compression, using some reasonable values. It is simple to plot both compression and tension strain on the same axis and, similarly, compression and tension stress using conventional negative values for compression. The different shapes of the two plots are easily seen. The slight curve in the elastic part of the plot is not an error; bone does not behave as a material that perfectly obeys Hooke's law. It can be seen that Young's modulus in tension is much greater than in compression by the steeper slope of the graph. In fact, the figures in this case are $16\,000\,\text{MN m}^{-2}$ for tension and $9400\,\text{MN m}^{-2}$ for compression, so compact bone is more elastic in compression than in tension. This is perhaps contrary to what might have been expected from a knowledge of the behaviour of collagen fibres not bound in bone. The second obvious difference is the strength. The ultimate strength in tension is about $120\,\text{MN m}^{-2}$ but for compression is around $170\,\text{MN m}^{-2}$. The value of mechanisms to convert tension to compression forces in bone becomes more obvious.

Energy storage capacity in bone

As already mentioned, the area beneath the stress–strain graph is proportional to the amount of strain energy. This energy is 'in store' while the bone is being stressed and a very small amount of the total available storage capacity is utilized physiologically. Thus, at each step there is a very slight elastic distortion of the lower limb bones, the energy being returned as the bone recovers. If the bone is much more strongly stressed, such as in a jump from a height, the bone distorts much more and is temporarily able to absorb much energy before fracture. A further effect that helps to prevent bone fracture is the fact that bones are stiffer and have greater energy storage capacity when the stress is applied very rapidly, which is the usual situation (Frankel and Nordin, 1980).

Any alteration of the bone structure, such as drilling a hole for some surgical procedure, will diminish the energy storage capacity very considerably. Experiments have shown decreases of 70% or even 90% in energy storage capacity for a few weeks after some procedures.

Bone adaptation

Bone is a living, changing tissue and is constantly being formed and removed. Consequently, it is able to respond over periods of days and weeks to changes in mechanical demands placed upon it. This response, enshrined in Wolff's law: 'bone is laid down where needed and reabsorbed where it is not', can alter the size, shape, structure, and importantly, density of bone. During prolonged immobilization of a limb, for example, there is a considerable loss of bone substance, which leads to a reduction in bone stiffness, strength and hence energy storage capacity. The extent to which this occurs obviously depends on the extent and length of immobilization. Experiments on monkeys, involving immobilization for two months, showed a threefold decrease in failure stress and energy storage of vertebrae tested in compression (Kazarian and von Gierke, 1969). Apart from immobilization, implanted metal attached to the bone, for stabilizing a fracture, may lead to local alterations in bone density, this being diminished where stress is taken by the metal and increased where stress is transferred from metal to bone. Striking losses of bone density have been found to occur in astronauts living for any length of time without the influence of gravity. The extent and rapidity of this change was somewhat unexpected in the early space experiments and illustrated the importance of everyday gravitational loads being continuously applied to the musculoskelatal system.

Effect of ageing and disease on bone

In the foetus, the cartilaginous tissue that will ultimately become bone is, of course, much more flexible; it has a Young's modulus of around 600 MN m^{-2}. This gradually stiffens as it becomes calcified during childhood to reach adult values about 30 times greater. This, coupled with their smaller size, accounts for the relative rareness with which fractures occur in children, despite frequent falling. In old age, there appears to be a decrease in the amount of bone tissue, which leads to a reduction in bone strength. This seems to be mainly a loss of energy storage, so that older bones tend to fail more readily under extreme stress.

While the loss of bone calcium appears to occur steadily from middle adult life onwards, it is under hormonal control and can sometimes be extreme, especially postmenopausally. This condition, called osteoporosis, leads to bone weakness, often in particular regions of cancellous bone, e.g. the upper ends of the femur and the humerus, the vertebrae and the lower end of radius. These areas then become prone to impacted fractures (compression of bone) and distortions, which can cause severe pain. The extent to which simple ageing contributes to this disease is disputed, but inactivity plays some part in allowing a lower initial bone density. It has been shown that bone density is associated with inactivity and that physical exercise can prevent or reverse this process (Rutherford, 1990).

Mechanical characteristics of soft tissues

The soft tissues of the body have rather different mechanical properties to those of bone described above. One similarity, however, is the fact that they are also more or less non-homogeneous. They consist of several materials with different properties, referred to as having 'phases'. This results in their stress–strain graphs being non-linear.

A generalized stress–strain graph for typical soft tissue is shown in Figure 2.11a. This general stress–strain interaction can be recognized in any self-manipulation of the soft tissues, bending a finger back into

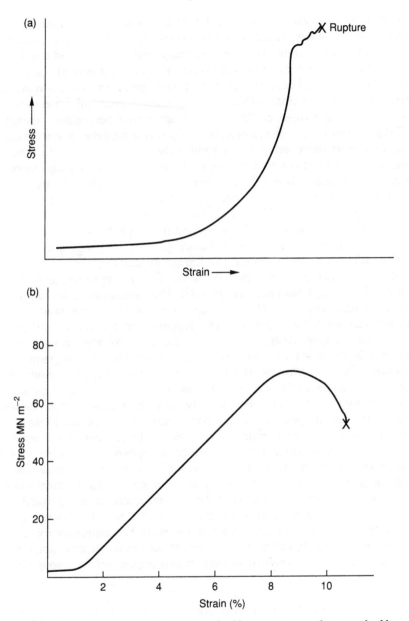

Fig. 2.11 Stress–strain graphs: (a) typical of human tissues; (b) typical of human tendon.

extension or twisting the external ear, for example. At first, much distortion occurs with little force but this becomes progressively less so quite rapidly and would require very great force to cause rupture. There is no evident plastic deformation until just prior to rupture. The actual deformity and force vary greatly with different tissues and at different sites. Cartilage is clearly much stiffer than loose skin. Much of the variation between tissues is due to the different properties and orientation of their components. Basic connective tissue consists of cells and a matrix. It is the matrix that confers the mechanical properties; it consists of fibres (collagen and elastic) and ground substance. Variations in the structure, quantities and orientation of these give the tissue its particular mechanical property. It is, therefore, pertinent to include a brief description of each.

Collagen fibres form bundles of various sizes, which interweave with one another. Unless stretched, they are irregularly sinuous or wavy. In tissues designed to resist stress in a particular direction, they lie parallel to one another in the line of stress. Microscopically they are seen to be made up of smaller microfibrils, which are themselves made up of filamentous tropocollagen molecules. These long (300 nm) protein molecules are each formed of three polypeptide chains wound in a triple helix. (Many amino acids are included but nearly one-third are glycine, with large amounts of proline and also hydroxyproline and hydroxylysine.)

These long tropocollagen molecules are firmly linked together with cross-bridges in a parallel manner but shifted longitudinally to one another by 67 nm (the so-called D-stagger, which accounts for the faint cross-striations visible microscopically). This repeated pattern gives a structure that is very strong in tension. The elasticity of collagen comes from straightening of the fibrils (see Fig. 2.11). The molecular arrangement is somewhat variable, allowing the formation of different types of collagen. (Type I is found in tendon and ligaments, whereas hyaline cartilage contains mainly type II; reticular networks of glands, lymph nodes, kidneys etc. are of type III, and are sometimes called reticular fibres.)

Elastin fibres are thinner than collagen fibres. Unlike collagen they are branched and yellowish in colour. They are composed of filaments of the protein elastin, which is made up of randomly coiled polypeptide chains that are cross-linked. This arrangement appears to allow greater elastic deformation to occur. Elastin contains several amino acids, particularly alanine and valine, as well as desmosine, which is unique to elastin. While elastin fibres are found in much connective tissue, the dermis for example, they are especially prevalent in some tissues such as the ligamenta flava of the walls of the aorta. Their presence accounts for the yellow colour of the ligamenta flava.

Mechanical properties of collagenous tissues

The collagenous or connective tissues of the musculoskeletal system and skin of the body are of three main kinds:

1. Tendons are concerned with transmitting tension force due to muscle contraction. Almost 80% of tendon tissue is made up of parallel collagen fibres, which are a little wavy when not stretched.
2. Ligaments are concerned with linking bones and limiting movement

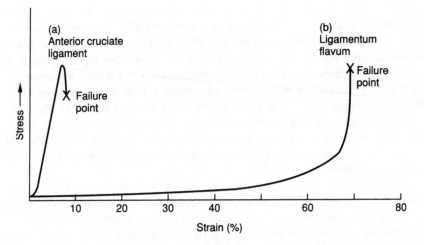

Fig. 2.12 Comparison of ligament with high collagen (90%) content (a) to a ligament with high elastin (60–70%) content (b).

between them. While some ligaments have many parallel collagen fibres, there are many in other orientations, depending on the function of the ligament.
3. The dermis, which has to be flexible and elastic in all directions, has its collagen fibres orientated apparently at random.

Mechanically, some of these tissues can behave rather differently from one another depending on:

1. The way the collagen fibres are orientated with respect to one another: if they are parallel, as in tendons, then they strongly and stiffly resist tensile forces (see Fig. 2.11b), whereas if they are in a network or mesh arrangement, as in the dermis, they allow a good deal of flexibility and elasticity in all directions.
2. The different properties of collagen and elastic fibres and their different proportions in the tissues: these different properties are well illustrated by comparing the typical stress–strain tension graphs for collagen fibres as shown by the anterior cruciate ligament, which is 90% collagen, with that of the ligamentum flavum which is 60–70% elastic fibres (see Fig. 2.12). It can be seen that, initially, collagen tissues elongate at very low stress – the 'toe' of the curve – due to the straightening out of the wavy fibres. Following this, there is an almost linear increase; it behaves in accordance with Hooke's law (see Fig. 2.11b), then gradual failure of the collagen bundles allows some plastic deformation to occur leading to final failure as many collagen fibres tear apart. This final rupture occurs after about 7–8% of tissue elongation, thus collagen tissue is elastic for about 3% or 4% of its elongation (see Fig. 2.12a and 2.11b).

Elastin fibres, as exemplified by the graph of the ligamentum flavum in

Figure 2.12b, behave in an entirely different way, allowing elastic elongation of some 50% of its length before a marked increase in stiffness occurs, leading to rupture at about 70% elongation. Pure elastin fibres elongate even further to nearly 200% before a sudden rapid increase in stiffness and rupture with no plastic deformation. (Young's modulus for elastin at $6\,\mathrm{MN\,m^{-2}}$ is close to that of rubber, but it should be noted that the stress–strain graph for rubber, and similar 'elastomers' as they are called, is sigmoidal, unlike that of elastic tissues.) Clearly, elastin fibres would be useful in tissues requiring considerable stretch and recovery that is rapidly repeated, such as the walls of the aorta or the parts of the larynx that vibrate during speech.

Ligaments and, particularly, tendons are stiff in that they take strong forces to provoke quite small elastic deformation in extension, which is a very useful characteristic for tissues that are connecting bones or connecting muscle to bone. For example, many repetitive activities, such as running (see Chapter 9), involve energy conservation by repeatedly stretching tendons as the foot takes the body weight on the ground and using the recoil to assist take-off. In this way the up and down movement of the body during running is not wasted energy. It is to some extent like using a pogo-stick in which the spring is compressed as the body moves down and bounces back to help the body rise again. As weight is put on one foot, the knee is forced into flexion and the ankle into dorsiflexion. Now, if the quadriceps and triceps surae contract isometrically, the stress stretches the quadriceps tendon and tendocalcaneus, which subsequently recoil, helping to push the body upward in the next step. Of course, the muscles must contract with the same force as that applied to the tendons but they are doing so largely isometrically, i.e. they do not change length very much, which is metabolically economical (see Chapter 4). At the same time, the joints of the arch of the foot are stretched and then recoil as the foot pushes off due to the elasticity of their ligaments, which also contributes to this effect. It has been calculated that adult men at marathon running speeds apply peak stress to their tendo calcanei of $53\,\mathrm{MN\,m^{-2}}$, causing approximately 6% elongation in the tendon (Alexander, 1992). This would account for some 18% of ankle movement, illustrating the very significant part played by this mechanism in running where there is little evident ankle movement. These figures for the tendo calcaneus are particularly high and calculations on other tendons have resulted in lower stresses at around 2% or 3% elongation in most situations. Nevertheless, the principle of storing energy in the elasticity of tendons and ligaments is widely exploited in the body. It is intuitively sensible to attach the force-generating muscles to the nearly rigid skeleton by flexible and strong elastic connections. Perhaps the best example of this mechanism is to be found in kangaroo hopping. These animals have a particularly massive gastrocnemius and tendo calcaneus and are able to exploit the mechanism described above so effectively that they can apparently increase their hopping speeds from less than $10\,\mathrm{km\,hr^{-1}}$ to over $20\,\mathrm{km\,hr^{-1}}$ without any increase in energy usage.

The tissues are not perfectly elastic. That is to say that after stretching they do not return all the energy in a mechanical form; some is lost as heat. Tendons are extremely efficient in this respect, returning some 93% of the stretch energy, hence losing only 7% as heat. This is as good as rubber but a little less than spring steel (Alexander, 1992).

Figure 2.12a illustrates what happens in ligament strains, sprains and ruptures. Minor ligament injuries produce pain but no clinically detectable abnormal joint motion. Thus the ligament has been stretched only to the initial part of the failure curve where some microfailure of collagen may occur, with perhaps minor neurovascular damage. More severe injuries involve clinically detectable joint instability, indicating rupture of some, but not all, collagen fibres due to stretching into the rounded top part of Figure 2.12a. The ligament is weakened. Very severe injuries involve complete joint instability, showing total ligament rupture. In fact, some fibres may remain to give the ligament an appearance of continuity (at operation) but it is unable to sustain loads.

Another variable that influences the strength and behaviour of ligaments is the rate of loading. Thus, rapid loading requires more force to rupture a ligament than a slowly applied force (Noyes and Good, 1976). This also occurs in bone, but not in exactly the same way, so that similar forces may cause ligament rupture or bone avulsion depending on the rate of force application. Loading ligaments and other collagenous tissues at relatively low stress for long periods of time can lead to two further types of change. First, what is called 'creep' may occur. This is a slow deformation of the tissue, which is most marked during the first 6–8 hours but can continue over very long periods. It apparently occurs mainly in the 'toe' region of the load deformation curve (Frankel and Nordin, 1980). Secondly, adaptive growth of the tissues will occur to adjust the length appropriately. This latter is seen in many pathological conditions in which unbalanced muscle pull or other forces act to overstretch particular ligaments, in genu recurvatum or scoliosis, for example. Attempts at therapeutic correction use these effects, e.g. the application of rigid or elastic splints in the treatment of talipes equinovarus. Much manipulative therapy is applied to ligaments and joint capsules with the expressed objective of stretching them. However, the speed with which an increased range of movement can occur suggests that the effect is neurologically or neuromuscularly, rather than mechanically, effected. Similarly, detailed investigation of the results of a four-week period of stretching the hamstring muscles (Halbertsma and Göeben, 1994) showed that the small increase of range achieved was due to increased tolerance to stretch and not due to any change in muscle elasticity. Ligaments and tendons, like bone, respond over time to the mechanical stresses regularly placed upon them. Thus the effect of repeated high stress levels is to promote greater strength and stiffness in the ligament and, conversely, the ligament weakens with reduced activity, such as during immobilization. Experimental work on primates has shown that two months' immobilization led to a reduction of the force needed to

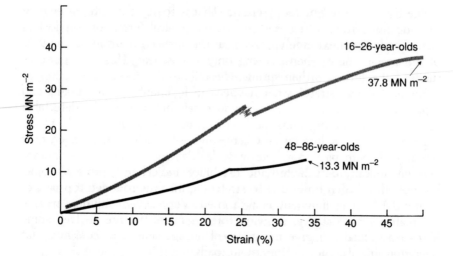

Fig. 2.13 Comparison of the stress–strain behaviour of ligaments from young and older humans (modified from Noyes and Good, 1976). (The kink in the line indicates the point at which some failure became evident.)

rupture the anterior cruciate ligament to 61% of that in controls. Recovery to near normal strength took a year (Noyes, 1977). This remodelling process is clearly quite prolonged and emphasizes the importance of a physical re-education programme after ligament or tendon injury.

Overemphasis on the mechanical properties of these tissues could be misleading for it must be remembered that both ligaments and tendons have extensive innervation. Thus, aside from pain, there is a considerable sensory input from these structures, contributing both to the proprioceptive control of joint movement and to protection. It may be that tension close to the limits may be allowable in tendons, e.g. in the tendocalcaneus noted above, because of efficient feedback from the golgi tendon organs. Similarly, ligaments influence the muscular control of joint movement by signalling their state of stretch.

The effects of ageing on ligamentous tissue (anterior cruciates) is illustrated in Figure 2.13 (modified from Noyes and Good, 1976), in which the stress–strain graphs from groups of older and younger humans are compared. It can be seen that the elastic modulus is greater in the young, being about 1.7 times that of the older group. An even greater difference is found in the maximum stress at failure, which is, as shown, nearly three times greater in the younger group. This study found an important difference in the mode of failure in that tendon rupture occurred in the younger group, whereas avulsion fracture of the cruciate ligament attachment tended to occur in older people. The change-over between these two modes of failure seemed to be around 50 years of age. Inevitably, the energy stored before failure is much greater in the young. This may be due partly to reduced muscular activity, but it may also be due to degenerative disease processes in the elderly. It is considered that tendons behave similarly and it may be noted that they rarely rupture in the young. The most frequent examples of such ruptures are associated with degeneration or repeated minor trauma, of the supraspinatus, long head of the biceps or extensor pollicis longus tendons, for example. Similarly, tendinitis is a frequent complaint in the middle-aged jogger.

Cartilage

The different varieties of cartilage have mechanical properties somewhat between those of bone and the soft tissues described above. These are largely due to the extensive ground substance associated with the fibres of the matrix. The preponderance of collagen or elastic fibres in white fibrocartilage and yellow elastic cartilage respectively, dictates the special properties of these types of cartilage. Hyaline cartilage is the most widely distributed type in adults, being found on almost all synovial joint surfaces and elsewhere.

The matrix of hyaline cartilage consists of collagen fibres and proteoglycan macromolecules. These latter consist of long-chain molecules. The whole arrangement is often described as a bottle-brush structure. It should be understood that there are many types and sizes of proteoglycan molecules present in cartilage as well as other protein molecules. Similarly, the collagen fibres, predominantly type II collagen, are of various sizes, with many smaller diameter fibres collectively forming a three-dimensional network.

These proteoglycan molecules are strongly hydrophilic. There are thus two separate mechanisms to account for the mechanical response of cartilage to loads. First, the presence of the solid matrix, mainly the collagen and, secondly, the contained water. This latter can move within, and be squeezed out of, the cartilage. In fact, cartilage may be considered like a strong elastic water-filled sponge. Common domestic experience of artificial sponges illustrates the features of such water-filled materials: first that light compression squeezes some water out but it takes a much stronger force to squeeze all the water out, and, secondly, that the force needs to be applied for some time to eject all the water. Both features depend on the permeability of the material. Domestic sponge material is infinitely more permeable than cartilage, i.e. the resistance to water moving through cartilage is very much greater.

The consequences of this are that rapidly applied forces, such as the compression of articular cartilage due to jumping, are resisted elastically as the force is transmitted throughout the tissue with no time for the water to move. On the other hand, prolonged pressure allows time for some deformation to occur as the fluid content can move from one part of the tissue to another. Indeed, it can move out of the cartilage altogether as occurs in articular cartilage, which is discussed in Chapter 6 in connection with joint lubrication. This feature of slow deformation under steady load with the exudation of fluid is the same as the creep described above for collagenous soft tissue, although the mechanism may not be the same.

It has been suggested that the higher fluid pressure in cartilage, as noted above, contributes to its elasticity in that some collagen fibres and proteoglycan molecules are already under elastic tension.

Much collagenous tissue is found in intimate relationship to muscle tissue as well as the typical tendons considered above – aponeuroses and perimysium – which behave mechanically in similar ways. Muscle tissue itself is separately described and its mechanical properties are considered in Chapter 4. Some other specialized collagenous and cartilaginous tissues, such as the intervertebral disc, are discussed later. Surface and lining tissues are further considered with lubrication in Chapter 6, as well as the factors that cause resistance to joint motion, some of which are pertinent to the structure and mechanical characteristics of the tissues discussed in this chapter.

3. Gravity, stability and balance: anthropometric considerations

Body movements are the result of many forces, both from within the body (pull of muscles and other forces), as well as from outside the body. At all times the human body on earth is subjected to a constant gravitational force. Due to this constancy, humans are accustomed to living in a relatively strong gravitational field to which all living organisms are adapted. The importance of a consistent gravitational force on the living human body becomes strikingly evident when it is removed or diminished as in space flight. Thus, astronauts in space need some mechanical help to maintain an upright orientation and tend rapidly to lose bone density and muscle strength if the state of weightlessness is continued for any length of time.

GRAVITY

Gravity is a force due to the attraction between two masses which is directly proportional to the product of the two masses and inversely proportional to the square of the distance between them. Thus:

$$F \propto \frac{m_1 \times m_2}{d^2}$$

Where the masses are small, the force will be small and hence is not easily detected, but if the total mass is large, the resulting force is large. Thus, an object the size of the earth has a very large gravitational effect on all other objects, notably on those near the earth, such as on its surface (see *Physical Principles Explained*, p. 177). This well recognized attraction between objects and the earth, in proportion to their mass, is described as the weight of the object. Since all objects on the surface of the earth are very nearly the same distance from the centre it is reasonable to use gravity to measure the mass of each object, weighing the object in kilograms. (Since the earth is not a perfectly spherical surface there are actually very trivial variations in weight from place to place.) Being a force, gravity due to the earth has direction – from any point on the surface to its centre – and is measured in newtons; it is $9.81\,\text{N}\,\text{kg}^{-1}$. In other words the acceleration due to gravity is $9.81\,\text{m}\,\text{s}^{-2}$. The concept of the weight of an object as a consequence of gravitational force is very important. Due to the constancy of gravitational force at the surface of the

Basic Biomechanics Explained

earth it is not unusual to use and compare forces in biomechanics in terms of their masses in kilograms or grams.

Centre of gravity

All parts of a body are influenced by gravity. Thus, for example, the two ends of a long rod of uniform density would be equally attracted to the centre of the earth, so that there is a balance point exactly in the middle of the rod on either side of which equal gravitational forces would act. The same applies in principle to any solid object of any shape so that there is a point in the centre of the mass of an object — the centre of mass — around which gravitational pulls due to all parts of the object balance one another. This is the point where the whole gravitational force on the object can be considered to act, and is called the centre of gravity. This point is not necessarily within the matter of the object. For example, the centre of gravity of a ring-shaped object of uniform density would be at the centre of the ring. For any rigid body, the centre of gravity always remains in the same place in relation to the body no matter what its orientation. Thus, the centre of gravity, somewhere in the middle of this book, remains in the same place within the book whether it is standing upright on a shelf or laid flat. When the objects considered are not rigid but can alter their shape — such as opening this book somewhere near the middle — the position of the centre of gravity changes (to near the middle of the spine in the case of this book). This situation applies to the human body, which is able to alter its shape by moving the body segments (see later). In a standing position with the arms at the sides, the centre of gravity is located approximately just in front of the second sacral vertebra in the mid-line of the pelvis. Altering the relative position of the body segments, say, raising one arm to the side, will alter the position of the centre of gravity because moving some of the body mass further to one side will shift the centre point of the total mass in that direction. Hence all body movement involves a constantly, often rapidly, changing centre of gravity, which necessitates constant adjustments as outlined below. A vertical line through the centre of gravity is called the *line of gravity* and will follow the changing position of the centre of gravity and will pass through different regions of a rigid object if its orientation is changed. Thus, a revolving wheel has the centre of gravity stationary at its axis or hub, but the line of gravity falls successively through different places as the wheel turns.

When one object is placed on another — supported on another — the gravitational force pressing down is counterbalanced by the reaction of the surface below pushing up, as discussed in Chapter 2. If the supporting force is not opposite to the gravitational force, the system is not in balance or equilibrium and movement results. In other words, the object placed on top falls over or falls off the one below. This is such a familiar experience that the underlying mechanism is often not fully considered.

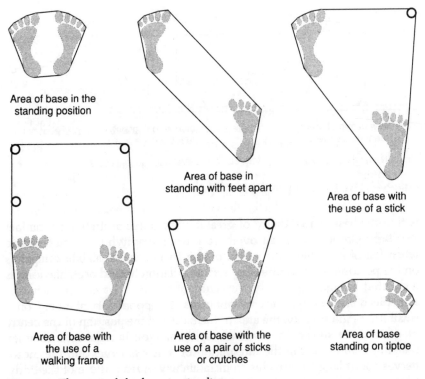

Area of base in the
standing position

Area of base in
standing with feet apart

Area of base with
the use of a stick

Area of base with
the use of a
walking frame

Area of base with the
use of a pair of sticks
or crutches

Area of base
standing on tiptoe

Fig. 3.1 The area of the base in standing.

The base of support refers to the area over which one object is supported by another, for example, the area enclosed by the four legs of a chair or table supported on the floor, or the area of this book placed flat on a table. If this book were stood on edge on a shelf the area of the base is now the smaller area of the bottom edge. In the standing position, the base of support of the human body is the area bounded by the contact points of the feet with the floor. Manifestly, moving the position of the feet and changing their area of contact will alter the area of the base, illustrated in Figure 3.1. Further, using a stick, a pair of crutches or a walking frame, as shown in Figure 3.1, will alter the area of the base. Sitting, kneeling or lying will provide a greatly increased base.

STABILITY

The stability of an object or body refers to the ease with which it can be unbalanced. This depends on the amount of energy needed to make the line of gravity fall outside the base of support and thus cause it to topple over. It takes more energy to move larger masses for greater distances. Greater stability is therefore found in objects of large mass with large bases and low centres of gravity, with their line of gravity situated well

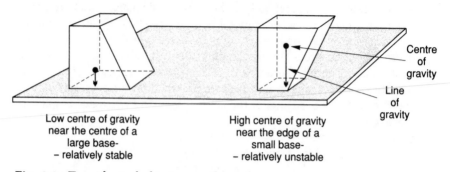

Low centre of gravity near the centre of a large base-
– relatively stable

High centre of gravity near the edge of a small base-
– relatively unstable

Centre of gravity

Line of gravity

Fig. 3.2. Two identical objects on a flat surface.

within the base. The stability of greater mass is demonstrated by the fact that light plastic bottles fall over easily when empty but are quite stable when full of liquid. For any given object, therefore, the stability depends on the position of the centre of gravity in relation to the base; this point is illustrated in Figure 3.2.

In the human body, the constant mass is supported in standing on a small base. Additionally, the area of the base and the position of the centre of gravity are subject to constant rapid changes. It requires a complex reflex system involving the integration of sensory nerves and the motor nerves controlling the muscles to maintain any given posture of the body. This is most evident in the upright posture but all others need similar control. A very large part of the human central nervous system is devoted to maintaining the balanced position of the large body mass during erect bipedal locomotion, which has evolved as a particular speciality in humans. Birds are also bipedal but have their centre of gravity below their hip joints, which improves their standing stability.

Upright balance

In order to maintain the upright position of any object with a relatively small base and high centre of gravity, such as the human body, it is necessary constantly to return the centre of gravity to a suitable position above the·base as it is disturbed. Even a slight disturbance of position causes the centre of gravity to move outside the base, increasing the torque or turning force so that it falls, accelerating, towards the ground. If a wooden pencil is placed upright, gently blowing on it will cause it to topple. In standing, deviation of the centre of gravity is constantly monitored by:

1. Sensory mechanoreceptors in the capsules and ligaments of joints, which provide information about their position and rate of movement.
2. Stretch receptors in muscles (muscle spindles), which give information on the amount and rate of muscle stretching.

3. The vestibular apparatus, including the semicircular canals found in the inner ear within the temporal bone of the skull, gives information of the motion of the head in all planes (see later).
4. Pressure receptors (exteroceptors) in the skin, which provide information about the amount of pressure on the skin of the soles of the feet in standing and the pressure on other body surfaces, such as the buttocks in sitting, or the palm of the hand when holding a stick or support rail.
5. The visual system giving information about the position of the body in relation to objects and surfaces that can be seen.

All this information is processed in the central nervous system — principally in the cerebellum and the brainstem — and signals are sent to skeletal muscles to contract appropriately to adjust the position of the body to maintain the centre of gravity over the base. This process involves unconscious prediction of body motion so that the adjustments are not merely responding to the existing body position, but arranging that the centre of gravity to base relationship is appropriate for subsequent movements, for example, the next step in walking.

Degree of stability

If much energy is needed to shift the line of gravity of an object outside its base, the object is said to be in *stable equilibrium*, whereas if a trivial force can cause it to fall, like the upright pencil, then it is said to be in *unstable equilibrium*. Notice that the difference is simply a matter of degree. In general, stability is associated with a large base and a low, centrally placed, centre of gravity, while instability is due to a small base and a high, eccentrically sited centre of gravity. These points are illustrated in Figure 3.2. If the disturbing force is removed before the line of gravity reaches the edge of the base then the object returns to the upright position. By having a curved base and a low centre of gravity, it is possible to push the object through nearly 90° while the centre of gravity remains within the base, as seen in rocking toys. If the applied forces do not alter the relationship of the centre of gravity to the bases, as occurs in a ball on a flat surface, then the object is described as being in *neutral equilibrium*.

Maintaining the equilibrium of the human body — balancing — is a fundamental and largely unconscious activity, as already noted. The ease of achieving it will depend on the factors affecting the stability of the particular posture to be maintained. Thus, the usual standing position can be rendered more stable by increasing the base by having the feet further apart, as shown in Figure 3.1. In sitting, stability is further increased, with a larger base and a lower centre of gravity, and prone or supine lying, with the largest possible base and a low centre of gravity, leads to the greatest stability. Conversely, standing on one foot or on tiptoe will diminish the area of the base and slightly raise the centre of gravity leading to a less stable position. In any of these postures, stability can be affected when the position of the centre of gravity is altered by moving part of the body. For example, raising the arms above the head will diminish stability.

Any object held or carried will influence the posture if its weight is a significant proportion of the body weight. This can be seen when a heavy bag is carried in one hand. The body is seen to lean to the opposite side and often the free arm projects from the side. Both actions are to keep the centre of gravity near the mid-line, as it would otherwise be displaced due to the weight of the bag. In this case the position of the centre of gravity over the base is being maintained by moving parts of the body, but sometimes the base is moved to keep it beneath the centre of gravity. Someone unexpectedly pushed from behind can be seen to take a quick step forwards to prevent themselves falling. This is an example of a reflex called a stepping reaction. Similar reflex actions include hopping reactions, which occur in situations where only one leg is free to move, such as when someone catches his/her toe going up steps. These reflexes are modified by many factors such as the nature of the surface and by learned balance cues.

To maintain an erect standing posture, continuous correction of the position is needed. This is achieved because sway occurs all the time, principally forwards and backwards, but to a lesser extent from side to side. This is not a fault in the system but a deliberate mechanism continuously to stimulate proprioceptors to provide a flow of information of the body position and hence allow immediate correction. It is a classical negative feedback, or servo, system and can be seen in the backwards and forwards sway of a standing subject. As forward motion occurs, the line of gravity moves towards the front of the area of the base – the toes – and reflexly provokes contraction of the calf muscles (principally the soleus, it is believed) to draw the body backwards so that the line of gravity now moves back towards the centre of the base, effecting relaxation of the calf muscles and allowing repetition of the cycle. This front to back sway is irregular and is combined with sway in other directions, which is controlled by other muscle groups so that the body moves continually and irregularly over the standing base. Standing on a force plate, which allows the centre of pressure of the standing base to be calculated and displayed, shows movement that is irregular in both time and direction in healthy subjects (see Fig. 3.3). If the eyes are closed, removing one source of information, the amount of sway tends to increase to compensate. Similarly, any interference with the normal reflex pathways causes increased sway, such as occurs in disease or to a minor and temporary extent in acute alcoholism. (The latter is an experience that has often been the subject of personal investigation by students and academics!) Not surprisingly, the amount of sway is greater in young children and decreases with maturation to a typical adult level, giving an average movement of the line of gravity of about 2.5 cm (Alexander, 1992). In old

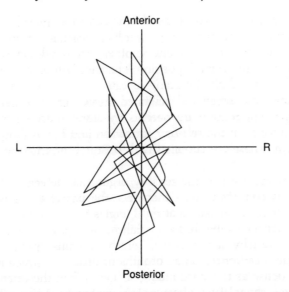

Anterior

L ——————————————— R

Posterior

Fig. 3.3 Typical track of the centre of pressure during normal standing on a force plate. Typical track wander in an area of about 2.5 cm diameter.

age, the efficiency of the mechanism declines and once again the amount of sway increases. Force plate recordings of this kind have been used to assess balance for diagnostic and therapeutic purposes.

As already noted, the position of the centre of gravity is changed with altered body posture. Thus, raising the arms above the head raises the centre of gravity and increases the amount of sway. Similarly, a crouching posture lowers the centre of gravity making the body more stable. Even in a fixed standing posture the exact position of the centre of gravity of the body is not easily specified. For one reason, the position of the abdominal contents varies with each breath depending on the position of the diaphragm. An approximate position for most adults is considered to be at the level of the second sacral vertebra in the mid-line and less than 5 cm behind the line joining the axes of the hip joints. This position, roughly in the centre of the pelvis, is true only in the standing position. Other postures will alter the position markedly. In some postures, for example, the backward arching of the modern high jumper, the centre of gravity may lie outside the body altogether. Naturally, the position of the centre of gravity varies a little in different individuals depending on physique. First is the different distribution of tissue volumes in men and women; the relatively larger pelvis and smaller shoulders of females gives, on average, lower centres of gravity in women. Similarly, babies and young children have relatively shorter legs than older children and adults, also giving lower centres of gravity. The different physiques among same sex adults, as discussed later, also leads to some differences in the position of the centre of gravity. As already mentioned, maintaining an upright posture requires a sophisticated control system, so the human nervous system has much of its capacity devoted to this end. Humans are singular in balancing a fairly heavy trunk on a pair of long lower limbs, each made up of a chain of bones balanced vertically on one another. Provided the column of bones can be kept in the vertical position – balanced on one another – the position is not particularly fatiguing because little muscular effort is needed and rapid movement is facilitated. However, in order to stay upright, constant corrections are needed by slight muscle contractions driven from neurones in the reticular formation and the vestibular nuclei of the brainstem. These are supplied with postural information as noted above.

The vestibular apparatus is the sensory organ that detects disturbances of equilibrium. It consists of two chambers, the utricle and saccule, and three semicircular canals arranged at right angles to one another, each in a different plane. Each chamber has a specialized area of hair cells with cilia projecting into a jelly-like material, which contains numerous small crystals of calcium carbonate called otoliths or otoconia, which are about three times as dense as the surrounding tissues. When the orientation of the head changes, the relatively heavy otoconia bend the cilia, stimulating impulses from nerve cells, whose sensory processes are connected to the base of the hair cells. At rest, there is a flow of impulses in most of the nerve cells, but bending cilia one way causes an increased number of impulses and bending them the other way decreases the number of impulses.

Because the cilia are orientated in many different directions, there is a different pattern of nerve impulses for all positions of the head in relation to the direction of gravity. This arrangement signals both the static head position and any linear acceleration. The semicircular canals contain fluid (endolymph), which tends to remain stationary, due to inertia, when the head is turned. The fluid thus deforms a sensory structure – the cupula – which signals the beginning of any rotation. Since the three canals on each side are approximately at right angles to one another, the start of all rotary motion (angular acceleration) is signalled. Thus, the canals give no positional (static) information but provide a signal of the start of angular motion, which will almost immediately affect body balance. They are said to have a 'predictive' function and are important in rapid movements. This latter point is illustrated when the semicircular canals of primates are compared; fast moving animals such as the gibbon have a larger radius of curvature of semicircular canals than slower moving species such as the gorilla. Human semicircular canals are distinctive in having larger anterior and posterior canals but a smaller lateral canal (corrected for body size). This is thought to be due to the need to monitor much vertical motion in bipedal walking. The size and shape of the canals in fossil skulls has been utilized to determine the extent of bipedalism and hence whether it is of great ape or hominoid type (Shipman, 1994).

Since the vestibular apparatus provides information of head position and motion, it is necessary that the brain should be provided with information of the position of the head relative to the rest of the body. This is given by proprioceptors, particularly by those of joints in the neck. Similarly, the relationships of other body parts are signalled to allow appropriate equilibrium adjustments to occur. As already mentioned, stretch receptors in the calf muscles would signal forward sway and proprioceptors in the ankle ligaments would inform on sway in all directions; additional information arises from pressure receptors (exteroceptors) of the skin.

The visual system makes an important contribution to maintaining a steady upright posture. If the eyes are closed when standing, a notable increase in sway occurs. Furthermore, vision seems to contribute to precision and co-ordination of postural adjustments. In normal standing, vision is not necessary for stability, self-evidently since, with a normal intact nervous system, balance is not lost in the dark or with the eyes closed. In fact, the basic mechanism for maintaining upright stance in humans is proprioceptive. It has been shown that a tilted visual stimulus does not alter body posture, although tilted body position does influence visual perception (Cody and Nelson, 1978). Having said this, it must be noted that, if the vestibular apparatus of both sides is destroyed, the visual system is able to compensate so that upright balanced posture can be achieved provided the subject is able to see.

While the basis of sustaining upright balance seems to be genetically fixed and naturally developed in the human nervous system – humans are 'programmed' to balance upright in the same way that they are preprogrammed to walk or talk – the quality of balance can plainly be improved by practice. This is seen in the gymnast, ballet dancer or high-wire entertainer. Similarly, the efficiency of upright balance may be diminished due to disease, disuse or old age. There is also a contribution from the higher centres, at least in predicting the direction in which balance may be lost, which is based on learned previous experience. This is evidenced by the unsteadiness felt by some people when stepping onto a familiar escalator which is temporarily stopped.

Disease mechanisms leading to instability

Patients with some disability in their balance system may suffer both from a proclivity to fall over easily and from the unpleasant sensation of unsteadiness. Any part of the reflex control system may be damaged, leading to different types of unsteadiness.

If disease occurs in the vestibular apparatus or vestibular nuclei it can lead to sensations of unreal movement called *vertigo*. This is sometimes described as being like the spinning sensation that persists in normal subjects for a while after alighting from a fast turning roundabout. This effect is due to a mismatch between different sensory inputs, with some indicating motion and others no motion. If the discrepancy is severe, it can lead to autonomic effects such as blood pressure changes, sweating and nausea. A similar mechanism accounts for the motion sickness that occurs in otherwise healthy individuals. If the vestibular apparatus of both sides totally fails, due to streptomycin poisoning, for example, or other injury, there is no vestibular input, so that rapid head movement, such as occurs in running or in a moving vehicle, causes apparent movement of the surroundings. For slow movements, input from other sources, notably the eyes, provides compensation. If there is a loss of proprioceptive information from the joints and muscles of the lower limbs, coupled with a loss of skin sensation in the feet, then unsteadiness will result. This can occur due to disease, such as multiple sclerosis, affecting the posterior columns (tracts of gracilis and cuneatus) of the spinal cord, which carry proprioception and touch sensations. The patient may adopt a stamping gait to try to increase the sensory input from the feet and legs and a wide base to counter the unsteadiness. (Such a gait was formerly often seen due to neurosyphilis in which the posterior tracts were selectively damaged.)

Disease involving the cerebellum, which is involved in the co-ordination or integration of sensory inputs controlling balance, can lead to evident instability. The unsteadiness and irregular overcorrection of leg and arm movements, coupled with the excess swaying gives an inco-ordinated gait, locomotor ataxia, often called cerebellar ataxia.

Injury or disease in the brainstem can also lead to various kinds of unsteadiness, including positional vertigo (in which specific head move-ment or posture causes vertigo) and sudden loss of upright posture ('drop attacks'). Many of these are due to some disorder causing reduced blood flow. Similarly, altered blood flow can cause unsteadiness as in the light-headed sensations that occur with postural hypotension. Although not an uncommon experience in normal subjects, on rising abruptly, for example, it often occurs in the elderly, because the efficiency of blood pressure control declines with age and is thought to be an important contributory factor to the cause of the falls that occur in this age group. Just as practice improves balance, lack of standing upright, such as occurs in those confined to lying for long periods due to illness, injury or surgery, leads to a loss of balance. In the otherwise healthy individual, the causes may be multiple but probably the main explanation is postural hypotension, which is rapidly rectified after a little practice. It may be noted that normal levels of consciousness are not necessary for efficient upright balance, as evidenced by sleep walking and epileptic or mildly concussed patients who walk apparently normally without conscious appreciation of what they are doing. On the other hand, some dizziness, but not usually overt instability leading to falls, may be psychologically induced.

Assessment of balance

Measuring disturbance of balance in any reasonably objective manner is not as simple a matter as might be thought. The degree of sway can be recorded from a suitable force plate as described earlier and shown in Figure 3.3. Such devices are flat, rigid metal plates supported on four piezo-electric transducers whose electrical outputs are integrated by a suitable electronic circuit continuously to record in some permanent form the position of the centre of pressure. Variations of the position of the centre of gravity are therefore recorded as the patient stands on the plate. This gives information of sway during standing, which is a reflection of balance competence.

Romberg's test was originally described in connection with tabes dorsalis (neurosyphilis). The patient is asked to stand with the feet together and eyes closed. If this provokes marked swaying, the test is positive and indicates damage in the posterior columns, vestibular system or cerebellum. Similar functional balance tests can be devised in which the posture and size of the base are specified and the patient is assessed as being able to maintain stability or otherwise. For instance, he/she might be asked to stand on one foot with the arms folded for ten seconds or with both feet together. Testing dynamic balance involves evaluating the ability to balance while performing some movement, say of the arms, or balancing on a moving base. The maintenance of balance disturbed by some outside force, an unexpected push, for example, or by distraction, can be assessed. These tests can be done first with vision and separately with the eyes closed (see Lane, 1969). Greater objectivity can be achieved by timing how long the patient can stand on one leg, which apparently correlates well with the general mobility of patients. A simple coding system to record the ability to respond to static, rotational and sagittal balance stresses has been devised (Gabell and Simons, 1982). This is especially applicable to elderly patients and provides easily measured and communicated information of their balance capabilities.

Body shape and size

What has been said concerning balance, stability and the centre of gravity of the body must be considered in the context of a wide variety of body shapes. It is perhaps necessary to point out first that there is no such thing as an ideal or even usual body size and shape. Normality lies in variety. In fact, body measurements – anthropometry – are normally (in the statistical sense) distributed. Adult north European males have an average standing height of 1 m 72 cm, with 90% of them being between 160 cm and 184 cm, with equivalent females having a mean height of 161 cm and 90% of them being between 150 cm and 172 cm. These figures are actually from Germany but figures for Britain, France and the USA are very similar (see Grandjean, 1980). As can be seen, and as is well recognized, there is considerable overlap between the sexes. Similar overlaps occur with all the other body measurements but the most striking differences between the sexes in respect of tissue bulk occur in the hips and shoulders. While the mean breadth of the shoulders in males (45 cm) is much greater than in females (41 cm) the breadth of the hips is very similar in the two sexes. It is actually larger in females in the German study from which these data are drawn (35 cm in males; 37 cm in females). In spite of the development of

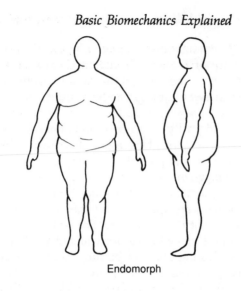

Endomorph

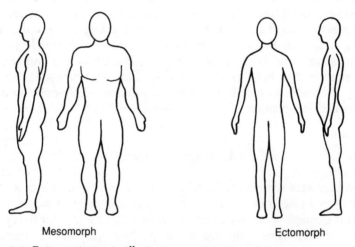

Mesomorph   Ectomorph

Fig. 3.4 Extreme types to illustrate somatotyping.

breast tissue, the relatively larger size of the adult female pelvis ensures that females have on average a somewhat lower centre of gravity than males.

Measurements of body weight show a similar distribution but are more dependent on variations in nutrition and other factors. Furthermore, these data are often taken from young adults, service recruits and students. Ageing tends to lead to a decrease in height and an increase in weight. The former is considered to be largely due to changes in the spinal column, with increased spinal curves, the latter to excessive nutrition. The American Government's *Vital and Health Statistics* (1966) found that people in the 45–65 years age group were 4 cm shorter, and heavier by

6 kg (men) and 10 kg (women), than their 20-year-old counterparts. Children show a similar spread of height, weight and physique appropriate to their state of maturity. In general, prepubescent children have their centres of gravity at approximately adult levels but younger children and babies have theirs at rather lower levels due to their relatively shorter legs. This factor assists the early learning of upright balance and walking. By five years of age most children have achieved virtually adult walking skills.

Beyond the simple division of adult body types into male and female, further classification of physiques has been attempted, initially by Hippocrates (as usual!) who distinguished short and thick from long and thin body types. In the early twentieth century, a three-group classification — pyknic, athletic and asthenic — was suggested. This basic idea was developed by Sheldon *et al.* (1940), who took and analysed many body measurements and concluded that physique could be classified by the extent of the contribution of each of three extremes. One extreme type was found to have large and well developed digestive organs, which are derived embryologically from the endoderm. Another extreme group had large well developed muscles, bones and circulatory system, derived from the mesoderm. The third had a large skin surface area; the skin and nervous system are derived embryologically from the ectoderm. He therefore coined the words endomorph, mesomorph and ectomorph to describe these extreme types (see Fig. 3.4). The contribution of each of these three to an individual physique was determined on a 7-point scale so that an extreme endomorph was classified as 7.1.1, and extreme mesomorph as 1.7.1 and an extreme ectomorph as 1.1.7. The detailed classification was based on some 17 measurements and fairly complex calculations, which produced about 76 somatotypes as they are called. (The full 343 categories ($7 \times 7 \times 7$) are naturally not available since people cannot be fat, thin and muscular all at the same time.) Of the 76 described by Sheldon, some 50 appear to be common. While the complexity of detailed somatotyping limits its use in clinical assessment, estimating the body type on this basis has proved to be helpful and is, apparently, reasonably accurate with a little practice (Karpovich, 1959). A single figure to give a rough idea of body build, particularly the ectomorphic component can be gained from an index derived by Karpovich:

$$\frac{\text{Body height}}{\sqrt[3]{\text{Body weight}}}$$

As might be expected, successful athletes are found to have a strong mesomorphic component. If the components are drawn diagrammatically, as shown in Figure 3.5, and the mean somatotypes of groups of outstanding athletes are plotted, it can be seen that endurance athletes tend to cluster to the ectomorphic side of the mesomorphic area, while weight lifters, shot and discus throwers group on the other. The above index should not be confused with the well-known Body Mass Index used

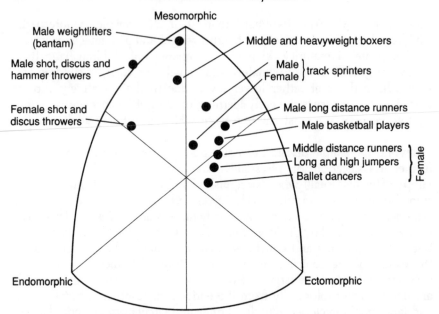

Fig. 3.5 Plot of mean somatotypes of various groups of top athletes (modified from Reilly and Secher, 1990).

to describe obesity. This is found from:

$$\frac{\text{Body weight in kg}}{\text{Body height}^2 \text{ in m}}$$

(a Body Mass Index greater than 25 is considered to indicate overweight and one greater than 30 to indicate obesity). Over a long time scale, the average human size and shape appear to adjust in response to environmental factors. Thus, over the past 150 years or so, improved diets have led to larger average body size in many developed countries. Adaptation to particularly hot or cold environments appears to have selected for particular physiques over many generations. Thus, the people of the Nile in Africa are tall with long, slim limbs, giving a large surface area relative to their mass, which enhances the effectiveness of sweating to lose heat in their hot environment. Inuit Eskimos, on the other hand, tend to be short and broad with a large mass and relatively small surface area to reduce their heat loss. While the broad pattern of body physique is genetically determined, it is also strongly influenced by eating and exercise habits, which particularly control the amount of body fat and muscle. Thus, the ultimate body shape of an adult is determined by many factors to which must be added age and disease. Obesity may be considered a disease. It has been found in England that some 8% of men and 12% of women were obese as defined by having a Body Mass Index over 30 (The Health of the Nation, 1992). Later figures (1994) suggest 13% of men and 16% of women are obese." The physical changes that occur

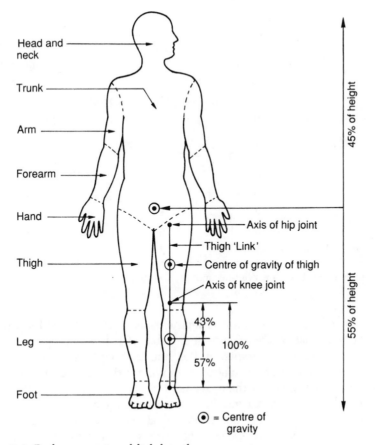

Fig. 3.6 Body segment and link lengths.

during childhood, pubescence and early adulthood, are well known and differ between the sexes. In old age, the recognized postural changes, decreased height and increased spinal curvatures, are associated with some general tissue loss. Diseases, both local and generalized, may markedly alter the physique.

Body segments

In order to analyse body motion it makes sense to consider the total mass of one body part moving on another. The term body segment is used in this connection to describe the whole of the tissues — bone, muscle, skin and all other soft tissues — in each separate body part. The functional body parts used to describe movement are: head, neck and trunk; thigh, leg and foot; arm, forearm and hand (see Fig. 3.6). The precise defining line between each segment is a matter of complex description, but the line of the flexure creases provides a reasonable approximation. While the size and shape of the body segments will vary greatly from one individual to

Table 3.1   Body segments

Body segment	% of total body mass	% of total body height	% of total body surface
Head	7	12 chin to apex	7
Trunk	50	35	34
Arm	3	17	4
Forearm	1.7 ⎫ 2.5	16	3
Hand	0.8 ⎭	10 wrist to fingertip	2.5
Thigh	10	25	9.5
Leg	4.5 ⎫ 6	25	7
Foot	1.5 ⎭	16 heel to toe tip	3.5
Foot height: talus to ground		3	

Approximate figures based on Williams and Lissner, 1962.

another, the mass and length of the segments as a percentage of the whole body are reasonably consistent; see Table 3.1 for the approximate relationships. Motion at joints in the **human body involves** complex gliding and sliding motions about a moving axis, but, for the simple analysis of motion, much of the movement of one segment on another can be described reasonably accurately in terms of angular motion around a fixed axis. A line through the proximal attachments of the collateral ligaments of the elbow, wrist, knee and ankle gives a satisfactory axis for flexion and extension of these joints. A line through the centre of the heads of the humerus and the femur is appropriate for the shoulder and hip for motion in a sagittal plane. Now it will be seen that these axes are not at the ends of their segments, i.e. the junction of the bones. A line joining the centre of the axis at each end of a segment is called a *link*. Thus, the arm and thigh segments are longer than the arm and thigh links, whereas the forearm and leg links are shorter. When the centre of gravity of the individual body segments is found it turns out to be at a specific point on the link line: 43% of the link length from the proximal axis and 57% from the distal. These relationships are remarkably consistent, as illustrated in Figure 3.6, not only for each limb segment but for the limb as a whole. Simple experiment will show that the height of the centre of gravity (at level of S2) above the ground in standing is also at about 55% of the body height. These consistent relationships give the best compromise for movement of the human body between the inertia of greater and more distal tissue bulk on the one hand and the fragility of long thin limbs on the other.

4. *Skeletal muscle contraction*

Human movement results from muscle contraction, therefore consideration of the way in which muscles function is central to an understanding of biomechanics. Muscle tissue contributes about 40% of total body weight. The term muscle contraction refers to muscle activity, which can occur whether the muscle is lengthening, remaining the same length or shortening. The term muscle is taken to mean a discrete anatomically described entity but it must be recognized that these do not necessarily function as independent units. Movement is often the result of contraction of a muscle group. On the other hand, individually named muscles may have parts that act in different directions or in different ways.

Muscles acting on the skeletal system usually cause or control motion at joints by reason of being firmly anchored to bones. The position of these attachments and their relationships to the axes of movement at the joints – the leverage – is crucially important in determining the force that can be exerted by that particular body part. This force – the external force – is thus the result of both the force exerted by the muscle and its mechanical arrangement in the body. The latter is discussed in Chapter 5, while this chapter is restricted to considering those factors that affect the force of contraction of the muscle itself. This is summarized below:

External force   – mechanical factors (Chapter 5)
                  – muscle force (Chapter 4)
                      – size of muscle
                      – type of contraction
                      – velocity of contraction
                      – length of muscle
                      – type of muscle fibres
                      – CNS control of muscle
                      – arrangement of muscle fibres (muscle architecture)
                      – effects of age, atrophy, hypertrophy

Before discussing these factors it is sensible to review, albeit briefly, the structure of muscle tissue and the way muscle contraction is brought about.

MUSCLE TISSUE

The basic cell of muscle tissue is the muscle fibre, which is a long, thin cylinder enclosed in a tough elastic sheath called the sarcolemma. Due to

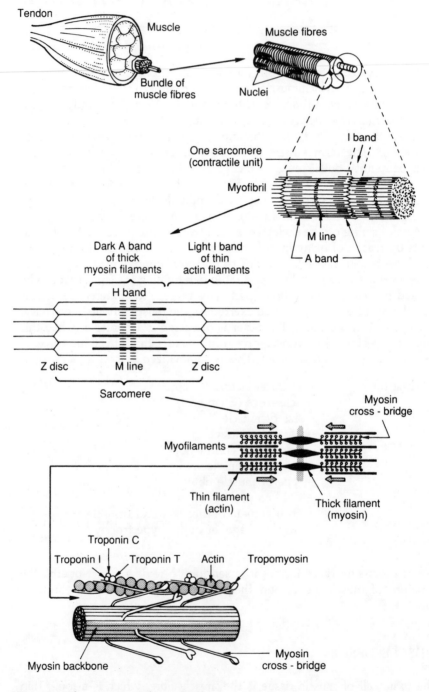

Fig. 4.1 The structure of muscle fibres.

its length (it can be several centimetres long with a diameter of 10–100 μm), it needs many nuclei, which are situated beneath the sarcolemma. The fibres are united to one another by connective tissue called endomysium and connected into bundles called fasciculi, which are enclosed by more connective tissue, the perimysium. Whole muscles are built of fasciculi enclosed in thicker connective tissue called epimysium.

Some 80% of the muscle fibre or cell is found to be made up of several thousand thin filaments called myofibrils, each about 1 μm in diameter. These are cross-striated in a regular pattern, the repeating unit being called a sarcomere. The visible bands and lines were given descriptive names which are customarily abbreviated to letters (see Fig. 4.1). While these striations have been seen for over 300 years (they were described in a letter from Leeuwenhoek to Robert Hooke in 1682) it has been the use of the electron microscope during the past 40 years that has elucidated their meaning.

The banded pattern is due to the overlapping of the protein filaments: thin actin and thicker myosin filaments, which interdigitate in such a way that each myosin rod is related to six thin actin filaments, each of which relates to other myosin molecules. The relationship is shown in Figure 4.1. The actin filament consists of a double string of actin molecules spiralling like two strands of a bead necklace twisted together. The myosin rod appears to be a set of two-headed molecules arranged so that the heads project in opposite directions and the tails form the backbone of the myosin rod. The heads form cross-bridges, which are able to link to and detach from the actin to draw one rod past the other, effecting muscle contraction. The control of this mechanism is by other proteins attached to the actin called troponins and tropomyosins, which are indicated in Figure 4.1

As well as the myofibrils, each muscle fibre contains numerous mitochondria for the production of the large amounts of adenosine triphosphate (ATP) needed for muscle contraction. Furthermore, in order to distribute the necessary nutrients and remove waste products from all parts of the cell an extensive transference system operates. This consists of the transverse tubule system, or T system, made up of infoldings of the sarcolemma into the cell; it connects to the sarcoplasmic reticulum whose tubules run parallel to and partly surround the myofibrils. Importantly, this arrangement allows transmission of electric charges from the muscle fibre membrane to all parts of the cell to ensure near synchronous contraction of all the constituent myofibrils.

MECHANISM OF CONTRACTION

When an impulse from a motor nerve stimulates a response in a motor end plate, an electric impulse passes through the T tubules, which 'unlocks' a calcium 'gate' in the sarcoplasmic reticulum. It does this by altering the

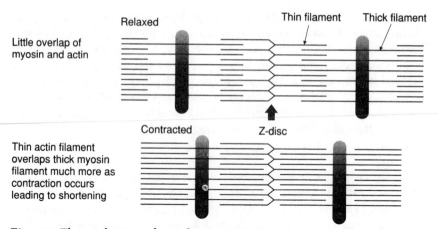

Fig. 4.2 The mechanism of muscle contraction

shape of a protein, which allows calcium ions to flood into the myofibrils. This alters the shape of the troponin molecules, which has the effect of allowing interaction between the actin and myosin. The myosin heads link to the actin, then alteration in the shape or angle of the myosin head occurs, which causes the thin actin filament to be pulled past the thick myosin for a distance of about 5–8 nm. These cross-bridges then release and reattach to the actin at another point. The whole cycle recurs repeatedly, pulling the two filaments past one another and, because of the opposite direction of the myosin heads, approximating the thin filaments to the centre of the A band thus shortening the whole sarcomere (see Fig. 4.2). The energy for this action is derived from the breakdown of ATP to ADP (adenosine diphosphate) and inorganic phosphate. It is believed that ATP is needed to effect the release of actin from myosin. As long as there is sufficient ATP and the levels of calcium remain high, the cross-bridges will continue to cycle. However, when the motor nerve stops firing, calcium release is prevented and, as troponin loses calcium, it reverts to blocking the interaction of myosin with actin so that the pull between them ceases. This complete sequence occurs very rapidly and, because there are many cross-bridges that do not act synchronously in an individual myofibril, a smooth contraction occurs.

CONTROL OF MUSCLE CONTRACTION

The events described above are initiated by nerve impulses arriving at the motor end plate. Each axon of a motor nerve branches as it enters the muscle so that each branch supplies an individual muscle fibre. The axon, its branches and the muscle fibres it supplies are collectively called a motor unit. Thus, a single nerve impulse from an anterior horn cell will trigger contraction in a group of muscle fibres at nearly the same moment ('nearly' because the fibres supplied are scattered throughout the whole muscle, hence having different lengths of neuronal pathway). This also helps to give an even muscle contraction. The number of muscle fibres supplied by a single axon varies, being few in muscles that are involved in very precise control, such as the eye muscles (6–12) and the lumbricals (about 100). In limb muscles, like tibialis anterior, several hundreds of muscle fibres may be innervated by a single axon and a few thousand in large limb muscle like gastrocnemius.

When a nerve impulse reaches the motor end plate it causes the secretion of acetylcholine into the gap between the nerve terminal and muscle sarcolemma. This provokes a change of conductance – the end plate potential – which causes the surrounding area of sarcolemma to depolarize with an abrupt influx of sodium ions. This potential is transmitted throughout the muscle fibre by the T tubules releasing calcium ions and causing a muscle contraction. This is a brief effect because acetylcholine is rapidly inactivated by acetylcholinesterase. To maintain continuous muscle contraction a stream of individual nerve impulses must arrive at the motor end plate to keep up the level of calcium in the muscle.

The tension developed in a whole muscle is the result of the combined effect of the muscle fibres scattered throughout the muscle that are contracting at the same time. Changes in tension are brought about in two ways. First, if an individual motor unit is fired by a nerve impulse, a single twitch of the muscle fibres occurs; a succession of impulses leads to a succession of twitches. As the frequency of nerve impulses rises, the resulting muscle fibre contractions merge together giving a continuous, stronger, tetanic contraction. This occurs because the nerve action potential is much shorter (at about 1 ms) than the resulting muscle twitch, which lasts for some 25–75 ms, so that at higher frequencies there is no time for the muscle to relax before the next stimulation. This is called summation. The second way of altering tension is by the number of motor units activated; the greater numbers obviously lead to greater tension.

FACTORS INFLUENCING MUSCLE TENSION

Size of muscle

The maximum tension that can be exerted by a whole muscle is related to its cross-sectional area, strictly to its physiological cross-section, since the fibres are often at an angle to the line of pull (see later). Various measurements have been made in humans (and animals) and muscles seem able to generate a maximum isometric force of between 30 and 45 $N\,cm^{-2}$ (newtons per square centimetre). When the muscle is being stretched, even greater forces ($50\,N\,cm^{-2}$) can be produced. It is hardly surprising to find that larger muscles can exert greater forces than smaller.

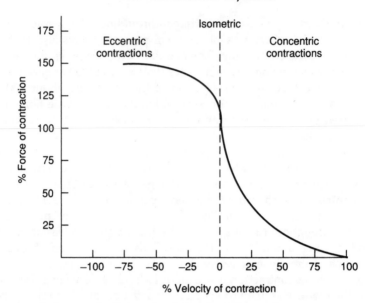

Fig. 4.3 A force–velocity graph of muscle. (Note – the axes are expressed as percentages: velocity of length change = 100% at zero force; force = 100% at zero velocity.)

Type of muscle contraction

Two different types of contraction were noted above. In isometric (same length) contraction, although muscle contraction occurs due to continuous cross-bridge cycling, there is no overall change in the muscle length. In isotonic (same tension) lengthening, the muscle is stretched out while contracting. Isotonic shortening, the most familiar type of muscle activity, is known as a concentric contraction and isotonic lengthening as an eccentric contraction. While these terms are familiar to and widely used by physiotherapists and physiologists, the latter term is, perhaps, not well chosen. However, while convergent and divergent might be better terms, concentric and eccentric are too hallowed by use to be changed and will be used in this text.

Velocity of contraction

The amount of energy generated by a muscle contraction can be seen both in the force of the contraction and in the rate or velocity of the contraction. It would be expected that higher velocities of concentric contraction would be associated with lower forces since the energy goes into shortening the muscle rather than producing force. This is clearly illustrated in Figure 4.3, which is a force–velocity plot in which both variables are expressed as percentages of their maximum. This point is also illustrated in Table 4.1. Notice that zero velocity is an isometric contraction and the force of this is taken as 100%. Even a low velocity, concentric contraction can be performed only at a markedly lower force than isometric contraction; the relationship is not linear. While the idea that greater force is associated with slower muscle contraction is reasonable and familiar – a heavier weight is lifted more slowly than a light one – the even greater force associated with eccentric contraction is not so self-evident. It must be realized that, as the muscle is being stretched by an outside force, there is passive resistance due to stretching of the elastic components, which is added to the active resistance due to cross-bridge cycling. Figure 4.3 shows that muscles exert their highest forces during eccentric contraction and their relationship with velocity is not the same as for a concentric contraction.

Table 4.1 Relative muscle force at different velocities

Velocity (% of maximum velocity)	Force (% of maximum force)
0.0	100
1.0	95
6.3	75
16.6	50
37.5	25
79.1	5
100.0	0

As a consequence, eccentric muscle activity is very much stronger than concentric. Thus any weight that can be lifted can always be lowered safely and easily. A great deal of muscle activity occurs as both eccentric and isometric contraction during normal physical activities (e.g. see discussion on walking in Chapter 9 and kangaroo hopping in Chapter 2).

Muscle length

The force with which a muscle can contract depends on its length at the time of contraction. This is illustrated in the length–tension graph of a whole muscle in Figure 4.4. Note that this refers to the muscle only; when moving bones at joints, the lever systems involved will modify this curve, as will be seen in Chapter 5. The equilibrium or resting length of the muscle is taken as 100% and, as the continuous line shows, isometric tension becomes greater as the muscle is stretched out. The reason for the non-uniform rise in tension is illustrated in the dotted lines, showing the increase in passive tension that occurs as the muscle is stretched and the change in active tension due to cross-bridge activation. The curve for

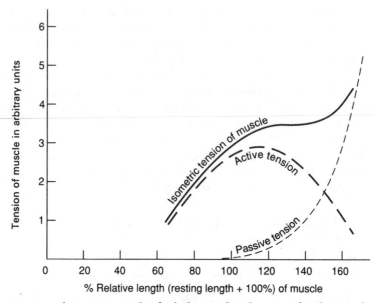

Fig. 4.4 Length–tension graph of whole muscle. The curve for the muscle is the sum of the active and passive curves (modified from Reilly *et al.*, 1990).

passive tension is reminiscent of those showing the tension changes in connective tissue with stretching, as in Figure 2.11a, which would be expected. The curve for active tension is due to the differing forces that can be generated with varying degrees of overlap between actin and myosin in the sarcomere (see Fig. 4.5). In this figure, the percentage of maximum tension is plotted against the sarcomere length in μm. As can be seen, the maximum tension (100%) occurs between 2.0 μm and 2.2 μm of sarcomere length, where the maximum number of cross-bridges can act between the actin and the myosin. As the sarcomere is stretched out, less and less overlap between the filaments can occur so that tension falls. Similarly, shortening beyond 2 μm leads, at first, to the actin filaments from each side overlapping and interfering with the cross-bridges and, ultimately, the myosin filaments abutting the Z discs, which leads to the rapid fall in tension. It was suggested above that the tension in muscles increases as they lengthen, due to stretching of the connective tissue, implying that only tissue outside the sarcomere is involved. However, it has been found that passive tension is generated within the myofibrils, due to a structural protein called connectin or titin, which connects the myosin filaments to one another (Lieber and Bodine-Fowler, 1993). Thus, tension is developed in the whole muscle by cross-bridge cycling, stretching both the structural protein of the myosin filament and other connective tissue, such as the tendons joining muscle to bone. These may be described collectively as the 'series elastic elements'. They are analogous to stiff springs. Similarly, the connective tissue ensheathing the muscle components, known as the 'parallel elastic element' can contribute tension

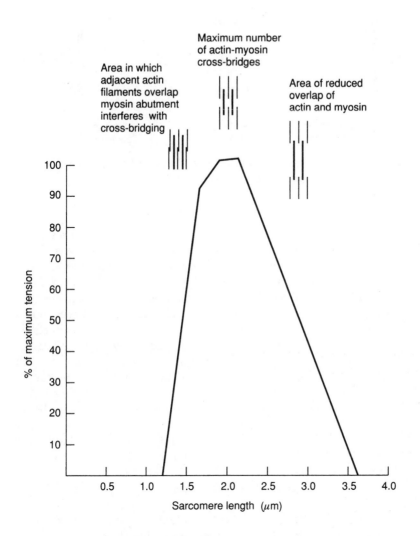

Fig. 4.5 Length–tension graph of a single sarcomere.

only when the muscle is being stretched. This idea is illustrated as a model of the system in Figure 4.6, which helps to illustrate what happens during isometric contraction in which no change in muscle length occurs, and yet the whole muscle is evidently doing work and using energy. Work (in joules) is done when the point of application of a force is moved, i.e. 1 newton moved 1 metre = 1 joule. Isometric contraction may, superficially, seem to violate this principle but, of course, the individual sarcomeres are shortening and stretching the series elastic elements so that a continuous set of length changes occur within the muscle as different groups of muscle fibres are involved.

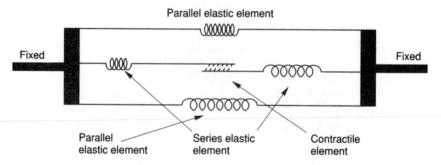

Fig. 4.6 Model of springs and contractile part to illustrate parallel and series elastic forces in muscle (modified from Buller, 1973).

Muscle fibre types

Muscle fibres are not all identical; the vast majority of human fibres can be classified as type I (slow twitch, red, oxidative fibres) and type II (fast twitch, white, glycolytic fibres). Type II are further divided into A and B, of which the latter is mainly glycolytic, while the former use oxidative phosphorylation as well as glycolysis and are thus intermediate in type. Nearly all human muscles have a mixture of muscle fibre types, but in most there is a predominance of one or other fibre type, which affects the contractile properties of the whole muscle. Type I slow twitch fibres are red because of large quantities of myoglobin, which is an oxygen-containing pigment like haemoglobin, and due to a rich blood supply. They take about 75 ms to complete their contraction, hence, they are slow but are able to maintain repetitive contractions for long periods before fatigue occurs. Type II fibres, on the other hand, fatigue more easily as their glycogen stores are utilized; they are rather wider and have more extensive neuromuscular junctions than type I fibres. They can contract about three times faster than type I fibres. These qualities make them appropriate for rapidly generating high forces for short periods. Thus, as a generalization, type I fibres are found mainly in postural muscles and muscle groups where their resistance to fatigue and ability to decelerate motion during eccentric contraction (because of the slower rate of cross-bridge cycling (Williams *et al.*, 1989)) are valuable properties.

Each motor unit appears to be made up of one type of fibre only. There is, however, evidence to suggest that the type of fibre is dictated by the frequency of nerve impulses applied and, further, that the fibre type can be changed by long term electrical stimulation (Salmons and Vbrova, 1969).

Nervous system control of muscle contraction

As noted already, muscle contraction is provoked by nerve impulses delivered via the motor units and the tension developed will be related to the number of motor units activated and the firing frequency. Both these contribute to the motor unit involvement, which can be assessed by measuring the electromyographic activity of the muscle. In general, increased muscle tension is associated with increased electrical output, as would be expected. During a submaximal contraction, although the tension may remain the same over a period of time, the electrical output – the motor unit involvement – tends to increase as muscle fatigue occurs. Thus, more motor units are involved to counteract the diminished tension due to muscle fatigue. Similarly, if the muscle is contracted to its maximum, the tension falls with fatigue but motor unit involvement remains at maximum. Further, more motor units are recruited for a given force of concentric than eccentric contraction (Berger, 1982). This would be expected from what has been described above.

Each motor unit is composed of only one type of muscle fibre, described above as I, IIA and IIB, so that there are at least three different kinds of motor unit each having characteristics commensurate with their muscle fibre type. It can be seen that the force and time course of a whole muscle contraction can be directed by the selection of appropriate types and numbers of motor units, as well as their firing frequency. It might be thought, since each motor unit is fired by a single nerve impulse, that all the muscle fibres would respond synchronously. This is not the case because of the way the muscle fibres are scattered throughout the muscle, with the result that the impulses will arrive at different times. Some fibres may also have a higher threshold and may not be triggered by a particular stimulus (Gowitzke and Milner, 1980). While the order in which motor units are recruited in a particular muscle contraction is a matter of uncertainty, it seems that, in general, the slower and weaker units are recruited first and the faster and larger fibres later. This orderly pattern of recruitment provides a means of regulating muscle force by proportional control. That is, the weak initial force is graded by weak increments and, as the force becomes larger, so do the steps by which it increases. This provides smooth force gradation when muscles contract. This is reminiscent of the way sensory discrimination (e.g. for loudness of sounds, brightness of light etc.) depends on the stimulus strength, the steps of discrimination being greater with a greater intensity of stimulus (Clamann, 1993). It must be realized that all motor units are not necessarily involved in a given muscle contraction. As some units are recruited, so others may drop out. Some appear to work only through a certain range of muscle tension.

In these ways the force output of a skeletal muscle can be controlled throughout an enormous range, typically more than ten thousandfold (Clamann, 1993). The relative importance of the two mechanisms for controlling gradation of force in muscle contraction – the number of motor units involved and the frequency of nerve impulses to each – is not well understood. Some evidence suggests that varying nerve impulse frequency accounts for force changes by a factor of only about five. While this indicates that motor unit recruitment is the more important mechanism, the relative importance of each is believed to depend on the muscle and its function (Clamann, 1993).

Muscle architecture

While the whole muscle is made up of similar sarcomeres, their arrangement in muscle fibres (see Fig. 4.1) and the arrangement of these muscle fibres are variables that affect the contractile properties of the whole muscle. Thus, muscle fibres may vary in length from millimetres to tens of centimetres. (Some fibres in the sartorius muscle may be up to 30 cm long.) Their diameters may also vary from about 10 μm to 60 μm (Williams *et al.*, 1989). The fibres are formed into muscle fasciculi with various orientations. Thus the fasciculi, and hence fibres and sarcomeres, may be arranged in a straight chain from one end attachment of the muscle to the other, in line with the direction the muscle is pulling. Alternatively, they may lie at some angle to the central straight line of the muscle. These arrangements of the fasciculi, parallel or oblique to the direction of pull, allow muscles to be classified by their architecture. Those with most of their fasciculi parallel to the direction of pull are straplike (e.g. sartorius), short straplike or quadrilateral (e.g. thyrohyoid), and straplike with tendinous intersections (e.g. rectus abdominis). In fusiform muscles, the fasciculi are very nearly parallel, converging to tendons at either end. Triangular muscles have fasciculi converging at one end, as the adductor longus. Where the fasciculi are angled between the parallel attachments, the arrangement is described as unipennate, as the flexor pollicis longus. The important bipennate arrangement (e.g. dorsal interossei) and that of multipennate muscle, such as deltoid, are shown in Figure 4.7a. Similar oblique arrangements of fibres and fasciculi occur in more complex ways in many muscles, such as the circumpennate arrangement of tibialis anterior.

The fundamental reason for these differences is that the excursion and velocity of muscle contraction is related to the number of sarcomeres in series. Hence, long straplike or fusiform muscles will have a great range through which they contract and can do so very rapidly. Muscle force, on the other hand, is proportional to the physiological cross-sectional area of the muscle, i.e. the number of sarcomeres in parallel not the cross-section of the anatomical muscle, as illustrated in Figure 4.7a. The various pennate arrangements allow more fibres to be applied to the moving tendon in any given muscle length, increasing the force generated but sacrificing the distance through which it can act (see Fig. 4.7b). Thus, the whole muscle can be structured to specialize in either rapid contraction through a large range or in force generation.

Of course, most muscles have structures that lie between the extremes. Since whole muscles are of different sizes it is possible to have muscles that exert high force due to a large number of fibres, while acting through a large range. If the graph of muscle force against muscle length is plotted for two muscles of identical mass, but contrasting architecture, the difference is evident, as shown in Figure 4.8. It can be seen that the muscle made up of long fibres with a small cross-section works through a greater range but with less maximum force than the short-fibred, large cross-

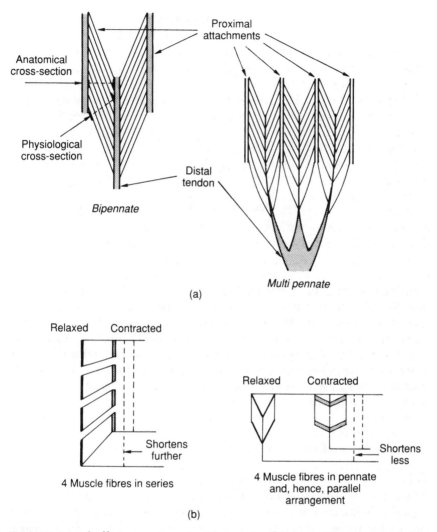

Fig. 4.7 Muscle fibre arrangements: (a) pennate; (b) shortening in series and in pennate arrangement.

section muscle. These graphs are hypothetical but illustrate the large differences that can result from variations in muscle fibre architecture. Measurement and dissection of human muscles show that there is a wide range of excursions and forces, some muscles more or less specializing in one or the other (Lieber and Bodine-Fowler, 1993). For example, sartorius, gracilis and semitendinosus appear to be suited to long and rapid excursions of low force because of their longer fibres and small cross-sectional area. This supports the suggestion that these three muscles, with their almost common distal attachment on the upper medial surface of the tibial shaft but attached proximally to three widely separated points on the pelvis, are concerned with balancing or stabilizing the pelvis and femur

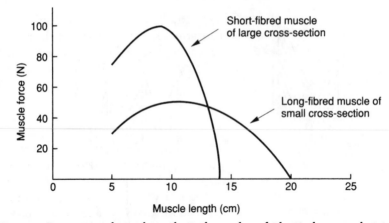

Fig. 4.8 Properties of two hypothetical muscles of identical masses but totally different muscle architecture (modified from Lieber and Bodine-Fowler, 1993).

over the standing tibia. On the other hand, the vasti of the quadriceps, and soleus and gastrocnemius appear to be specialized force-producing muscles due to their opposite characteristics of short fibres and large cross-sectional area. This is a consequence of their antigravity functions. The actual angle of the pennate fibres to the tendon determines the force and range (see Chapter 1) and resolution of the forces. The range is proportional to the fibre length multiplied by the cosine of the angle of attachment to the tendon.

Other factors affecting muscle force

Sex

While it is well recognized that adult males have greater muscle strength, on average, than females, the reasons are complex. The average adult male has nearly twice the strength of an equivalent female in the shoulder musculature but only about a third more in the hips and legs. This is partly due to the greater development of the shoulders in men but it is also a consequence of the greater average size of males (see the heights and weights noted in Chapter 3). When muscle strength is expressed per unit body weight, some of this difference is lost. Nonetheless, a substantial difference remains so that, on average, women have some 60–80% of the strength of men. The difference is considered to be due to hormonal action, with testosterone enhancing muscle and connective tissue development, and the greater amount of muscle tissue formed in males. It should be emphasized that such descriptions are only applicable to the average of large numbers of subjects; large variations occur between individuals and groups. In fact, many of the studies comparing muscle strength are limited to particular, often highly selected, groups, which may not be generally representative. However, grip strength (which is a reasonably universal activity) has been found, in a number of studies, to show females exerting 75–80% of male strength. There is also considered to be a cultural effect in the groups studied, which influences the expectations and hence muscular activity of growing boys and girls (Berger, 1982).

Age

Growth and maturation are naturally associated with increasing muscle strength and, as would be expected, strength correlates closely with body weight. Up to the age of about 11 years, the strength of children increases, boys being only slightly stronger than girls on average. During adolescence, the increase is markedly greater in boys, leading to the mean adult differences noted above (Berger, 1982). During adult life, muscle strength seems to reach maximum at between 20 and 30 years; from then on it follows a slow decline so that by age 65 it has fallen to about 80–85% of its maximum. This general pattern has been deduced from a number of studies of age related changes but it must be understood that other factors, notably the amount of exercise taken, may alter this pattern so that in some instances adult strength remains almost constant throughout much of middle adult life.

Exercise and nutrition

The proteins of which muscle tissues are formed are constantly being broken down and replaced so that adjustments of muscle quantity occur in response to increased or diminished use. In the former case, hypertrophy occurs in which muscle bulk increases. Exactly how this increase occurs is a matter of uncertainty, although it is considered that muscle fibre hypertrophy occurs rather than an increase in cell numbers (hyperplasia). There is evidence that in humans muscle strength, endurance and fibre type can be altered by appropriate exercise. In general, it seems easier to change metabolic muscle properties (i.e. improve endurance), rather than increase contractile force. While muscle force can be greatly increased in untrained individuals by moderate exercise regimens, this need not necessarily be associated with a muscle tissue increase, at least at first. This suggests that the immediate increase in muscle strength is due to neurological changes – motor learning – but exactly how it occurs is unclear (see also Chapter 5). Naturally, real muscle hypertrophy can only occur with adequate nutrition. During starvation, especially on a low protein diet, the opposite occurs in that the subjects metabolize their own skeletal muscle tissue to provide nutrients and energy. This loss of muscle tissue – muscle atrophy – also occurs as a consequence of disuse. This effect is strikingly demonstrated by patients who have had limbs immobilized for any length of time; the loss of tissue is evident after removal of the fixating cast.

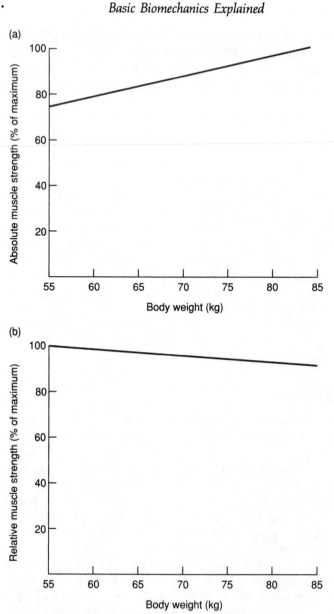

Fig. 4.9 Body weight and muscle strength relationships: (a) absolute strength; (b) relative strength (modified from Berger, 1982).

Hormonal and genetic

There are marked differences between individuals, some have a particularly well developed musculature, i.e. the mesomorphs, noted in Chapter 3. Thus, there is a considerable genetic component in the ability to develop strong muscle that is linked to the secretion of hormones; the effect of testosterone was noted above. Thyroxin and androgens, as well as steroids, contribute an anabolic effect.

Relationship of body weight to muscle strength

It has already been noted that muscular strength correlates closely with body weight, but, of course, it is not a perfect correlation because of the varying amounts of other tissue, notably fat, that contribute to total body weight. However, if a more or less homogeneous group is considered, such as the college age males on which the data for Figure 4.9a is based, then the averaged relationship is regular as shown. In this group of young adults the lightest, at about 57 kg, had about three-quarters of the average strength of the heaviest, at around 84 kg. If these data are expressed as relative strength per kilogram of body weight, it might be expected that there would no longer be a difference and all would be equal. It turns out, however, that the light subjects are relatively slightly stronger, i.e. the situation is reversed (Fig. 4.9b). Why lighter bodied men should be relatively a little stronger is not apparent, but it could be due to the fact that endomorphs with more fat and less muscle tissue in their body build are more represented among heavier subjects.

This chapter has been concerned with some of the features of skeletal muscle that determine the force with which it can contract. In the next chapter, the forces exerted on, and by, body segments due to muscle contraction are considered.

5. Parallel force systems: application of muscle forces to body segments

Systems in which forces are parallel to one another but not in line were described in Chapter 1 as parallel force systems; it was noted that they tend to produce rotary motions. Such systems are seen in all kinds of mechanical devices as well as in the human body.

The simplest situation is to consider a rigid object, a bar, for example, which is pivoted at some point, well known as a *lever*. If a force is applied on one side of the pivot, it provokes a force in the opposite direction in the part of the lever on the other side of the pivot. Classical and familiar examples are the beam of a beam balance, a see-saw (teeter-totter in USA) or the crankwheel of a bicycle. In the case of the beam balance, the length of the arms on each side of the pivot are the same so that weight (mass acted on by force of gravity) in each weighing pan can be directly compared. If they balance, the forces, and hence the masses, on each side must be equal. In the case of a see-saw this need not be the case since a light child may balance a heavier playmate by sitting further from the pivot, fulcrum or axis. Thus, the turning force, or *torque*, in a parallel force system must take account of both the magnitude of the force and the perpendicular distance of the force from the pivot. This is referred to as the *moment of force*. It is found by multiplying the force by the perpendicular distance between the line of action of the force and the axis of rotation. Thus the 40 kg, 12-year-old, who has been bribed or bullied into playing with a 20 kg younger sibling, would need to sit half as far from the axis as the position of the lighter child to give balance (see Fig. 5.1a). These distances are often called the *lever arms*, the distance between the input force or *effort* being called an *effort arm*, and that between the output force or *load* or *weight* being called the *load arm* or *weight arm*.

The concept of input and output forces for a see-saw is not particularly relevant, but if a long steel bar is being used to lift a heavy drain cover (Fig. 5.1b), the value of being able to lift a heavy load with less effort is apparent. In this example, a small force acting through a large distance at the input is altered to a large force through a small distance at the output, with the heavy drain cover being lifted. The work done – force × distance – is of course identical at both ends of the lever. The ratio of the load force to the effort force is proportional to the ratio of effort arm to load arm and is sometimes called the *mechanical advantage*:

$$\text{Mechanical advantage} = \frac{\text{Load}}{\text{Effort}}$$

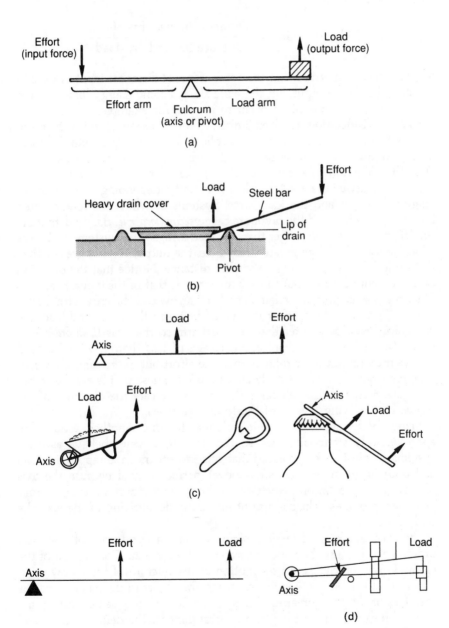

Fig. 5.1 Lever systems: (a, b) first order lever – balance; (c) second order lever – power; (d) third order lever – speed.

Notice that this is a force ratio, so that, if the output force is the larger, the mechanical advantage will be greater than one and vice versa. The movement at the two ends of the lever can be described as the *velocity ratio*. Since the two ends move different distances in the same time, the velocity ratio is the ratio of the distance moved by the effort to that moved by the load:

$$\text{Velocity ratio} = \frac{\text{Distance moved by effort}}{\text{Distance moved by load}}$$

It has been suggested that the work (force × distance) input is exactly equal to the work output, but there are always some energy losses during motion: friction at the pivot or air resistance, for example.

So far, consideration has been limited to the situation in which the pivot or axis lies between the points of application of the effort and the load. Such systems, which are sometimes described as *first order levers*, serve to alter the direction of motion of the applied force and may provide a mechanical advantage greater or less than unity, depending on the relative lengths of effort and the load arms. Systems in which the load is sited between the effort and the pivot are called *second order levers*. By definition, the effort arm must be longer than the load arm, so this system must have a mechanical advantage greater than 1, i.e. the output force is greater than the input, but acting through a smaller distance. Notice that the direction of movement of the output force is the same as that of the input. Examples of such systems include the familiar wheelbarrow and the crown top bottle opener. Similarly, if the effort is situated between the pivot and load, the effort arm must be shorter than the load arm so that this *third order lever* must always have a mechanical advantage of less than 1, with the load always moving further and faster than the effort but in the same direction; a simple example is of a drop latch for a door. These points are illustrated in Figure 5.1c and d. In all cases the arrows indicate the direction of the *motion* of a moving lever, not the force (see later).

Many body segments move relative to one another around an approximately stationary axis, so that the rigid bones behave as lever systems. It must be emphasized that this is very much an approximation and body segment movement is never perfectly axial because the axis moves during rotation. Analysis of body mechanics in these terms, however, provides valuable insight into an understanding of the way the body functions.

The vast majority of lever systems within the body are of the third order type just described and illustrated in Figure 5.2a. Contraction of the elbow flexor, brachialis, causes motion at the fulcrum of the elbow joint, which results in elbow flexion, i.e. raising the object in the hand as well as the weight of the forearm. Other examples of the same system are abduction of the arm at the glenohumeral joint by the deltoid muscle and raising the lower limb by flexing the hip due to contraction of the iliopsoas. By siting the muscle attachment close to the centre of rotation

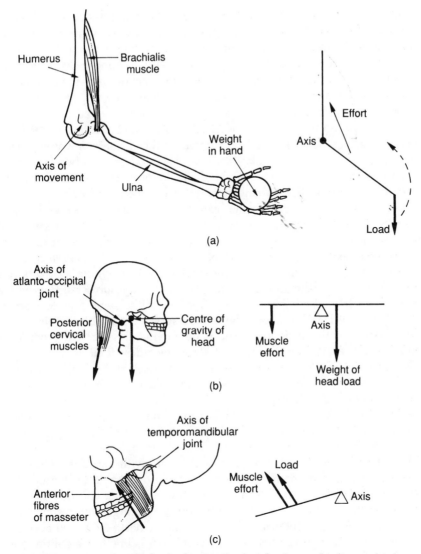

Fig. 5.2 Lever systems in the body: (a) third order lever; (b) first order lever; (c) second order lever.

of the joint, as in this system, the benefits of great speed and range of the limb extremities are achieved, with the active muscle contracting through only a small range but with great force.

In some balancing situations, the first order lever system is found. Flexion of the head at the atlanto-occipital joint is controlled by the posterior cervical muscles as the head tips forwards. This is often seen during travel — especially on evening commuter journeys — when the passengers' heads nod forward in sleep, to be abruptly pulled upright as the jolting of the train wakes them. In full extension, the centre of gravity of the head lies behind the axis so that the flexor muscles now act to pull the head forward (see Fig. 5.2b). The same leverage system works to balance the trunk at the hip joints, the gluteus maximus and hamstrings acting to oppose flexion, and the iliopsoas to oppose extension, in standing. Note that the same muscle, iliopsoas, acting over the same joint, works in a different lever arrangement as noted above, depending on whether the limb is moving on a fixed trunk or vice versa.

Within the body there are few situations in which second order lever systems are evident. The anterior fibres of the masseter muscle usually pass in front of the back molar teeth, so that food crushed between these teeth as the mandible is elevated lies closer to the axis of the temporomandibular joint than the anterior part of the muscle.

Lever systems in one plane can be considered in several ways, depending on the reference point chosen, the axis, about which movement occurs. Thus the movement of plantarflexion, with the ankle joint considered as the axis — as in plantarflexing the foot against some resistance by contracting the triceps surae — then the whole foot acts as a first order lever. If the foot is on the ground with the subject sitting with a weight on the bent knees, then contraction of the same muscles can be seen to cause rotation about the metatarsophalangeal joints, raising the load applied at the ankle joint. This is now evidently a second order lever system. (This latter arrangement is sometimes described as occurring in the standing position, but clearly causing the heels to rise with the line of gravity behind the axis of the metatarsophalangeal joints will cause the body to fall over backwards.)

Complex chains of lever systems can readily be seen in all kinds of familiar objects, such as movable desk lamps in which the weight of the lamp and reflector on a long arm is supported by a strong spring on a short lever arm. This kind of arrangement, with muscles acting like springs, is found in many situations in the body. It will be recalled that lever systems can be used to alter both the magnitude and direction of a force. This is also effected with continuously rotating lever systems, such as gear wheels and pulleys; the bicycle crank wheel was noted above. In these cases, the rope or chain moves with what is in effect a continuously rotating first order lever with identical effort and load arms (see Fig. 5.3a). If one side of the rope is considered as the input or effort and the other the load, then such an arrangement can only change the direction of the applied force. Such direction-changing pulley-like arrangements are found in the body in situations where tendons change direction, in synovial sheaths, across joints such as the fingers and toes, or in other situations such as the long head of biceps at the shoulder, peroneus longus around the cuboid bone or extensor pollicis longus on the dorsal surface of the radius.

Pulley systems can also be used to alter the force in the way illustrated in Figure 5.3b, in which the fixed end of the rope becomes the pivot and the load is attached to the axle. In this system, the effort arm is always twice the length of the load arm or vice versa, so that the system can act

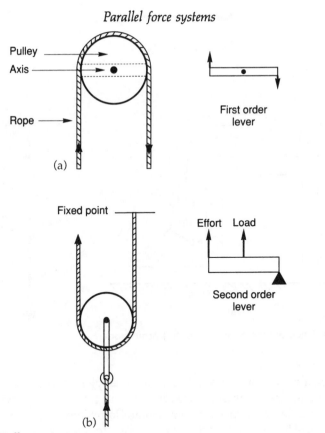

Fig. 5.3 Pulley systems.

either as a second order type lever with a mechanical advantage of 2 or a third order type with a mechanical advantage of $\frac{1}{2}$ depending on which rope applies the input force.

Rope and pulley systems are widely used in rehabilitation devices to provide resistance to body motion, e.g. 'multigym', 'Westminster pulley system' and simple weight and pulley circuits. They are also utilized to provide steady traction forces and control reciprocal movement. In all these, the central purpose is to alter the direction of forces (in one plane) so that, for example, a weight acting vertically downwards can be used to provide resistance to motion in a horizontal or any other direction. Some devices also utilize the force-changing capability of pulley systems. In order to achieve a mechanical advantage of greater or less than 1, multiple pulley systems are used.

FINDING FORCES

As it is usually impossible to apply direct measurement to muscle tension or joint compression, it is therefore necessary to estimate these from forces that can be measured.

Basic Biomechanics Explained

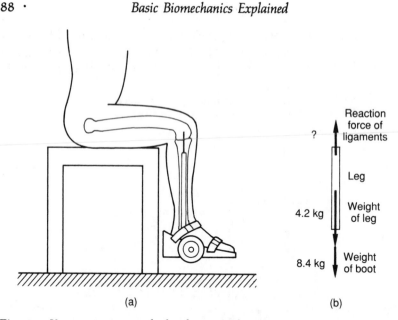

Fig. 5.4 Knee extension with the de Lorme boot.

Taking a very simple application as an example, weights are attached to the foot with the thigh supported in a sitting position to provide strong resistance to knee extension as a rehabilitation exercise for the quadriceps muscle (see Fig. 5.4a). It might be of interest to know what force, beyond the weight of the leg, needs to be supported by the knee joint ligaments while the leg is dependent and the muscle relaxed. This can be ascertained from the diagram in Figure 5.4b. These are sometimes referred to as free body diagrams and are used to describe the forces involved. If a 70 kg (154 lb or 11 st) man, lifting a total weight attached to the foot (de Lorme boot and weights) of 8.4 kg (18.5 lb) is considered, the forces can be shown: from Table 3.1, the mass of the leg and foot is approximately 6% of the 70 kg, i.e. 4.2 kg; since the leg is supported only from above and is stationary, then the ligaments must exert a reaction force that is equal and opposite to the total force acting downwards:

$$(4.2\,\text{kg} + 8.4\,\text{kg}) \times 9.81 = 123.6\,\text{N}$$

Thus, the ligaments are resisting a force three times the usual weight-free condition, which leads to the suggestion that this position should not be continued for prolonged periods and the weight and foot should be supported between lifts.

Notice that this is a linear force system, as described in Chapter 1, and also that the forces are all proportional to the masses (weights) so that the same answer would be arrived at if weights were considered. The steps taken in this simple example can be formalized and the principles applied to many force analysis problems in biomechanics. Since a static situation is being considered, the system is in equilibrium, so the sum of all forces, or moments of force, acting on the object or body part being considered must be zero. So, for forces in one plane, three conditions must be met:

1. All vertical forces must summate to zero;
2. All horizontal forces must summate to zero;
3. All moments about any axis must summate to zero.

These can be formalized as three simple equations (Σ – sigma – means 'add up' or summate):

$$\Sigma V \text{ (vertical forces)} = 0$$
$$\Sigma H \text{ (horizontal forces)} = 0$$
$$\Sigma M \text{ (moment of force)} = 0$$

In the example above there were only vertical forces to consider and it was obvious that they acted in opposite directions, weight and body part downwards and reaction force of ligaments upwards. It is conventional to call downward acting forces positive and upward acting forces negative. Horizontal forces to the right and clockwise moments are taken as positive, while horizontal forces to the left and anticlockwise movements are negative. Thus the example in Figure 5.4 can be written as:

$(4.2 \times 9.81 \, N)$ + $(8.4 \times 9.81 \, N)$ – $RN = 0$
(mass of leg × acceleration)   (mass of weight × acceleration)   (reaction force of ligaments)

so

$$RN = 123.6 \, N$$

As another example of finding vertical forces, it is assumed that the two children (one of 20 kg and one of 40 kg) on the see-saw in Figure 5.1 are balancing with the beam of the see-saw, which weighs 15 kg, horizontal. What reaction force must be acting at the axis? (For simplicity, the acceleration due to gravity is taken as $10 \, m \, s^{-2}$.) Note the direction of the forces is considered, not the direction of the movement.

$$+200 \, N + 400 \, N + 150 \, N - RN = 0$$

so

$$RN = 750 \, N$$

If the load of rubble and the wheelbarrow in Figure 5.1c is assumed to have a weight of 60 kg and a combined centre of gravity 40 cm from the axis of the wheel, what force (f) is needed to support the barrow from a point on the handles 1 m from the axle and what reaction force (R) would be exerted at the axle? Taking moments about the axis of the wheel:

$$+600\,N \times 0.4\,m) - (F\,N \times 1\,m) = 0$$
$$\text{(clockwise)} \qquad \text{(anticlockwise)}$$

so

$$F = 240\,N$$

This is equivalent to lifting a 24 kg weight at the handles. Considering the vertical forces:

$$+600\,N \quad -240\,N \quad -RN = 0$$
$$\text{(downward) (upward) (upward)}$$

so

$$R = 360\,N$$

Thus, 36 kg is supported through the axle and via the wheel by the ground.

While providing resistance to muscle contraction, it is of consequence to know something of the force acting at the joint involved. Thus, if the elbow is flexed at 90° and a physiotherapist provides a force of 40 N at the wrist to resist isometric contraction of the elbow flexors at the distances shown in Figure 5.5, what force will the elbow flexors be exerting and what will act to compress the elbow joint? (The elbow flexors are, for convenience, being considered as only the biceps brachii and its attachment on the radius.) The weight of the forearm is ignored.

$$\Sigma H = 0$$

Hence:

$$+\,40\,N \,-Fb\,N + Fj\,N = 0$$
$$\text{(to right) (force of) force of joint}$$
$$\text{biceps to \quad compression to}$$
$$\text{left) \qquad right)}$$

Taking moments about the joint axis:

$$\Sigma M = 0$$

Hence:

$$+\,(40 \times 25) \,-(Fb \times 5) = 0$$
$$Fb = 200\,N$$

Substituting this value into the horizontal forces equation above:

$$+40\,N \,-200\,N + Fj\,N = 0$$
$$Fj = 160\,N$$

Thus, the compression force on the joint is quite considerable and would be proportionally even greater with larger forces. The force applied to the

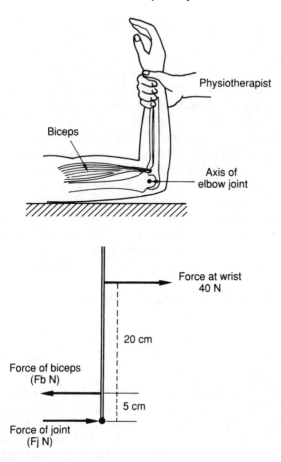

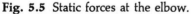

Fig. 5.5 Static forces at the elbow.

wrist above is in no way exceptional. The mean maximum isometric elbow flexion force of young adult males has been found to be nearly ten times this value, at about 382 N (Williams and Lissner, 1962). Now, suppose it is considered advisable to reduce the compression force on the joint while retaining the same muscle force. Thus, if the force applied by the physiotherapist is increased to 100 N and applied closer to the elbow, just 10 cm from the axis, then the same procedure shows:

$$+ (100 \times 10) - (Fb \times 5) = 0$$

so that

$$Fb = 200 \, N$$

and

$$+ \, 100 \, N \, - 200 \, N + FjN = 0$$

so that now

$$Fj = 100 \, N$$

Thus, the joint force has been reduced by nearly 40% (37.5%) without decreasing the muscle force.

As an example of use in a clinical situation and to illustrate the way different axes may be utilized, consider a patient strengthening very weak quadriceps isometrically. The patient lifts the whole lower limb a few centimetres off the supporting surface, keeping the knee straight, with a de Lorme boot and weight totalling 3 kg attached to the foot. It is intended that the patient should continue the exercise at home using a weighted cuff that fits around the leg above the ankle. If the centre of gravity of the weighted boot is 50 cm and that of the cuff is 30 cm from the axis of the knee joint, what weight of cuff (X) will be equivalent to the weighted boot? Figure 5.6 illustrates the arrangement. The isometric quadriceps, contraction acting at its tibial attachment, must oppose a turning moment due to the weight of the leg and foot acting at the centre of gravity of the limb segment and that due to the weight of the boot. Since the former remain constant, it is only necessary to consider the latter. Thus:

$$3 \text{ kg} \times 0.5 \text{ m} = 1.5 \text{ kg m} = X \text{ kg} \times 0.3 \text{ m}$$

so

$$X = 5 \text{ kg}$$

therefore, a 5 kg cuff is appropriate.

Notice that what is being considered here is the proportional torque about the axis of the knee joint but, in order to lift the leg, the hip flexors will have to shorten. What difference will the cuff make to the force they must generate? Again the effect of the weight of the lower limb will be the same in both circumstances. If the axis at the hip is assumed to be 40 cm from the axis of the knee, the boot has a turning force proportional to:

$$3 \text{ kg} \times 0.9 \text{ m} = 2.7 \text{ kgm}$$

and that of the cuff

$$5 \text{ kg} \times 0.7 \text{ m} = 3.5 \text{ kgm}$$

Thus, the hip flexors will need to exert a greater force with the cuff than with the boot, but not in proportion to the figures given above because the constant weight of the lower limb would be the most significant part of the load being lifted. For a 70 kg patient, the lower limb weighs 11.2 kg (16% from Table 3.1). With the centre of gravity close to the axis of the knee at 40 cm from the hip, the turning force of the lower limb would be proportional to:

$$11.2 \times 0.4 = 4.48 \text{ kgm}$$

hence, 7.18 kgm with the boot and 7.98 kgm with the cuff.

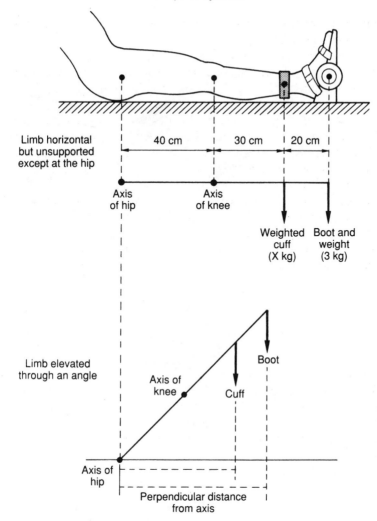

Fig. 5.6 Isometric quadriceps exercise with weights applied at two different sites.

This example can be used to illustrate further effects that occur. So far, only static situations or, as in the case above, very little motion, has been considered. If, however, the lower limb was raised to a significant degree, the perpendicular distance would alter between the centre of gravity of the limb and the weight, and the axis at the hip. In the extreme, at 90°, the weight of the limb and any added load would be directly over the axis of the hip, so that no turning force would be exerted. Thus, as the limb is raised, the distance – and hence torque – diminishes in proportion to the cosine of the angle of the limb with the horizontal at the hip joint (see Figs 5.6 and 5.7).

A second point is illustrated by the fact that the direction of pull of neither the hip flexors nor the quadriceps is at right angles to the long axis

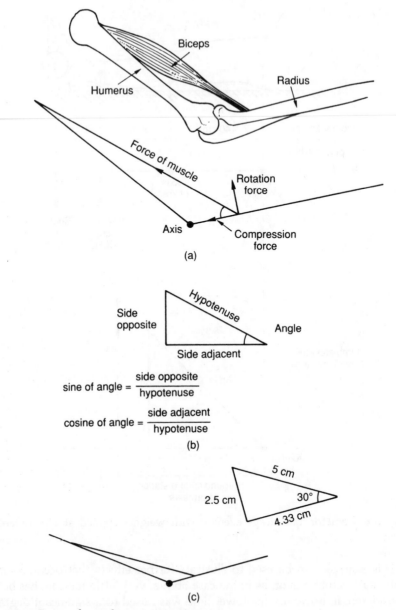

Fig. 5.7 Force of muscle in various directions.

of the limb segment. Hence, the forces exerted by these muscles are only that proportion that acts in the appropriate direction. It was described in Chapter 1 how forces can be resolved into components. The simplest case, which is appropriate in this and many other instances, is that of two forces at right angles to one another. This allows the formation of right-angled triangles to effect algebraic solutions to simple problems.

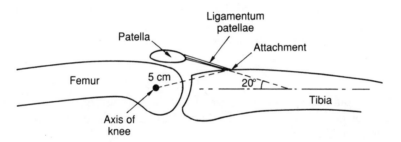

Fig. 5.8 Section through the knee joint.

In the example shown in Figure 5.6, it is obvious that the knee is being held in extension by the quadriceps muscle acting through the ligamentum patellae. The line of action of this force is at an acute angle to the long axis of the tibia, so that only a proportion of this force will act at right angles to the tibia, the rest acting to press the tibia against the femur at the knee joint. This situation occurs in most joints. The position of the elbow in relation to the biceps muscle was specially chosen in Figure 5.5, so that the muscle acted at right angles to the bone to avoid this complication. More usually, muscles act at an acute angle to the long axis of the bone as shown for the brachialis in Figure 5.2. (In all these examples, the more forceful action of the biceps in causing rotation of the radius (supination) is being ignored and only the flexion component considered.) The proportions of the muscle force that act at right angles to and in the long axis of the bone are the same as the proportions of the two sides of a right angle triangle when the hypotenuse is at the angle of the muscle pull (see Fig. 5.7a and b). Thus, a knowledge of the angle of pull and the force of the muscle will allow the turning and joint compression forces to be deduced. The sine of the angle is equal to the length of the side opposite the angle divided by the length of the hypotenuse (Fig. 5.7b). It can be seen that, at larger angles, the side opposite will be a greater proportion of the hypotenuse. Similarly, the cosine of the angle is the length of the adjacent side divided by the length of the hypotenuse and will become smaller at greater angles (see Appendix B).

As an example, if the angle that the active muscle makes with the bone in Figure 5.7c is $30°$, (sin $30° = 0.5$ and cos $30° = 0.866$), then the force acting to flex the elbow is 50% of the total muscle force, whereas that compressing the joint surface is 86.6% of the muscle force. It should be remembered that the muscle force exerted, not the energy expended, is being discussed and that it is the *square* of the hypotenuse of a right angle triangle that equals the sum of the squares of the other two sides. This makes reasonable the fact of the addition of the component forces being greater than the original. In Figure 5.6, if it is assumed that the ligamentum patellae makes an angle with the tibia of $20°$, as shown in Figure 5.8 (sin $20° = 0.342$), then the quadriceps will need to provide a force some three times the rotational force to keep the leg straight in extension. The distance between the axis of the knee and the attachment of the ligamentum patellae is about 5 cm (see Fig. 5.8), i.e. the moment arm of the quadriceps muscle pull (P). Thus for a 70 kg subject:

$$-(P \times 5) + (4.2 \times 21) + (3 \times 50) = 0$$

(quadriceps pull (P) × 5 cm + the weight of the leg and foot (4.2 kg) with its centre of gravity assumed to be 21 cm from axis of knee + 3 kg boot, 50 cm from axis of knee).

The muscle pull, P, is, therefore, 47.24 kg or 463.4 N (47.24 × 9.81).

Now, because of the 20° angle of pull of the quadriceps, the total force exerted must be much greater, as shown above. Thus:

$$\frac{463.4 \times 100}{34.2} = 1354 \text{ N}$$

Thus, the quadriceps muscle is contracting with a force of some 1354 N in this example. While this may seem large it is a small proportion of the maximum possible force (of about 5000 N) that can be generated by the quadriceps. It will be recalled that forces of some 30–40 N cm^{-2} can be produced, so that the large cross-section of the quadriceps provides a very large force.

It is perhaps now clear why the strength of muscle has been considered in two parts, in Chapters 4 and 5. What is regarded as muscle strength from a clinical point of view is actually due to torque. Activities such as walking, moving the arms or kicking a ball, are all manifestations of torque in the musculoskeletal system. The two aspects of force generated by muscles (Chapter 4) and relationships between muscle attachments and joint axes (this chapter) are being considered separately.

So far, only the static situation of the isometric quadriceps contraction of Figure 5.6 has been considered, but it is clear that during joint motion the angle of the muscle would change. This is evident in Figure 5.7, in that, if the elbow were flexed further, the angle between the muscle and the radius would increase, allowing a greater proportion of the muscle force to act as a turning force. Similarly, as the elbow extends, the reverse occurs leading to a greater proportion compressing the joint surfaces together and less acting as a turning force. This compression force is sometimes described as 'wasted' because it does not contribute to the joint motion being considered, but this is a misconception because it contributes to joint stability, which is a necessary part of joint function. In the case cited above, it can be seen that, if the elbow is in full extension, the head of the radius will tend to be distracted away from the humerus, so that increased joint compression will usefully counteract this. Thus, the maximum torque that can be exerted on the limb segment depends on the angle of the muscle pull and hence varies throughout the range of motion as the segment moves at a joint. This is no simple matter to calculate, since many muscles (described as single muscles anatomically) have extensive attachments, which pull in different directions, and joint motion is never exactly axial and is often highly complex. These difficulties can partly be resolved by considering the directions of the individual fascicular units that make up the muscle and calculating the change of position of the axis during joint motion. It will also be apparent that the relationship of muscle attachments and joint motion will dictate how far the muscle can lengthen or shorten. This should be considered in connection with what was said about muscle architecture in Chapter 4. In general, muscles with long fibres tend to have large movement or they are two-joint muscles, i.e. features adapted to allow a large range of rapid movement and low force. Those with large cross-sectional areas generally have short moment arms (Lieber and Bodine-Fowler, 1993), but this is not always so. Many muscles seem to have architectural structures to compensate for their anatomical relationships. These considerations have led to a classification of muscles depending on the position of their attachments, giving a predominance of one of three kinds of activity (MacConaill, 1949). Thus, some muscles, such as brachialis, act strongly to produce angular movements and were called 'spurt' muscles. Others, acting along the shaft of the bone to cause joint compression, such as brachioradialis compressing the elbow joint with the humerus fixed, were called 'shunt' muscles. The third component, not so far considered, is that of rotation around the long axis of the bone called the 'spin' component, hence 'spin' muscles. This spin component is most evident where muscle action produces almost pure rotary motion, e.g. the pronator quadratus. While less obvious, almost all muscles act to produce rotation in some degree.

From the multiplicity of factors described in this and Chapter 4, it is evident that the maximum torque will vary over the range of motion of a joint. The maximum isometric torque at different points in the joint range can be measured to provide a graph to show the relationship. The two factors that mainly dictate the shape of these curves are first the degree of stretch (length) of the muscle and secondly its angle of pull. Thus, in the case of elbow flexion from the fully extended position, at first the muscle is fully stretched and, as it becomes shorter during flexion of the joint, so it is able to exert less force. However, as has been shown, relatively little torque can be exerted in full extension but it becomes greater and greater as the elbow flexes, bringing the angle of pull of the muscle closer to a right angle with the forearm. Thus, the combined effect provides the greatest torque around 90–95° of elbow flexion, with lower torque at full extension, because of the ineffective angle of pull, and at full flexion where the muscles are too shortened to generate much force (see Fig. 5.9a). It must be understood that it is the whole group of elbow flexor muscles – brachialis, biceps, brachioradialis, pronator teres and the other muscles attached to the common flexor attachment on the medial epicondyle of the humerus – that are involved. As can be seen in Figure 5.9, this pattern is not universal to all joints. It would seem that muscle length has the greater effect (see Fig. 5.9c and d). It should be emphasized that the graphs of Figure 5.9 are in some degree approximations and may be altered if the

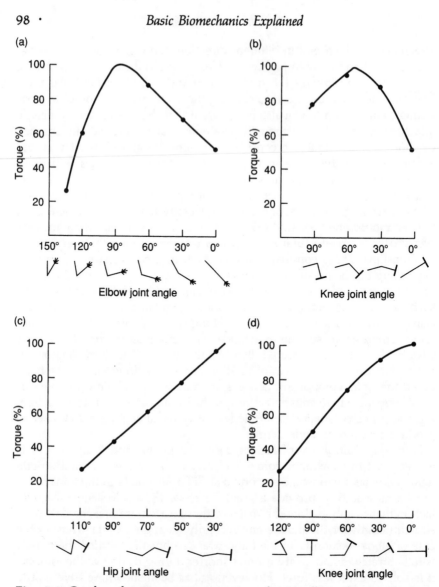

Fig. 5.9 Graphs of torque against joint angle: (a) elbow flexors; (b) knee extensors; (c) hip flexors; (d) knee flexors (prone).

subject is tested in a different position. They show the torque expressed as a percentage of the maximum for comparison, but the actual forces would differ greatly between the muscle groups. While it was noted that these were based on a series of maximum isometric values, it is perfectly possible to provide curves based on isokinetic testing, which have essentially the same shape. In isokinetic testing, the maximum dynamic force is measured with the movement occurring at a constant speed (see later). From what was noted in Chapter 4, it would be expected that the isometric torque would be the greater, which is the case (the faster the

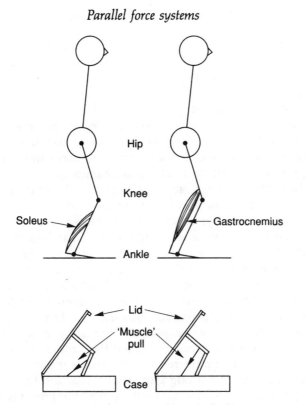

Fig. 5.10 Muscles acting on limb segments to which they are not attached.

isokinetic velocity of motion the lower the torque). The shape of the resulting curve, however, is very similar.

In such testing situations, the movement is isolated to a single joint but in most real life situations the limb segments interact with one another and with external forces. This can result in muscle being able to act on limb segments to which it is not attached, and about joints which it does not cross. To see how this might occur, consider the soleus acting on the tibia with the foot on the ground. If the trunk is relatively fixed (due to its inertia, for example), then the knee joint will be extended, so also will the hip joint (see Fig. 5.10). Even more surprising is the idea that, under some circumstances, two-joint muscles may act to move limb segments in the opposite direction to their recognized anatomical actions. Thus, the gastrocnemius may act to extend the knee in upright standing rather than flex it (Zajac, 1993). To see how these effects can occur, consider the jointed rigid bracket used to hold open the lid of a case, as illustrated in Figure 5.10. Because both ends of the bracket are hinged, the pull on the lower arm, like the soleus, will force the knee of the bracket into a straightened position, i.e. extension. Similar effects occur when the upper arm of the bracket is pulled on by the 'gastrocnemius' which would act to bend the 'knee' if it were free at the upper end. This is a single example, but it must be clear that the way in which a muscle acts can change from task to task and from moment to moment. The forces exerted on a body segment by a particular muscle will vary depending on the other forces acting on that segment and the previous force changes, that is, the force dynamics.

To illustrate further the complexity of muscle action in normal activities, the role of two-joint muscles may be considered. It has already been noted in Chapter 4 that some two-joint muscles, sartorius, gracilis and semitendinosus, are remarkable for having long fibres and relatively small physiological cross-sectional areas. These characteristics suggest a control function throughout a large range, perhaps in stabilizing the pelvis over the tibia. Other two-joint muscles of the lower limb, rectus femoris and gastrocnemius, have large cross-sectional areas and are clearly able to produce great force. During standing jumps, it has been found that the single-joint muscles, gluteus maximus, the vasti and soleus, provide the main propulsive energy, while the gastrocnemius and rectus femoris contribute just prior to take-off, acting to 'fine tune' the co-ordination of the jump (Zajac, 1993). The nature of the 'fine tuning' is further elucidated by studies that show that during jumping and locomotion there is a transfer of mechanical energy between joints by means of two-joint muscles. This concept is sometimes called the 'tendon action' of muscles and can be illustrated with reference to the rectus femoris. If the hip joint is being extended by the strong gluteus maximus and the rectus femoris contracts isometrically – i.e. it does not shorten, but prevents lengthening – then some force of hip extension is used to cause knee extension; the rectus is, therefore, acting like a tendon. Thus, energy can be transferred from hip joint to knee joint by the two-joint rectus femoris. It has been shown that during the push-off phase of running and jumping the 'tendon action' of two-joint muscles (rectus femoris and gastrocnemius) transfers energy from the proximal to the distal joints. During the shock-absorbing phase, energy is transferred from distal to proximal joints (Prilutsky and Zatsiorsky, 1994). This arrangement enables the larger, and hence more forceful, proximal muscles to contribute both to push-off and to absorbing energy in landing. If the distal muscles only were involved they would need to be larger, giving the distal segments much greater inertia and leading to slower motion. The advantages of lower inertia in body segments can be seen in the long slender legs of deer and horses, in which the power is provided by bulky muscles close to the body, giving very rapid movement for fast running.

MUSCLE FATIGUE AND ENDURANCE

A well recognized, but not fully understood, feature of muscle activity is the fatigue that occurs and leads to decreased muscle strength. It is common experience that a maximum isometric contraction can only be sustained for a very short time; around five seconds is usual. Static muscle contractions that are less than maximal can be sustained for proportionally

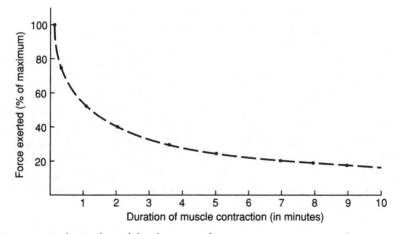

Fig. 5.11 Relationship of the duration of maximum isometric muscle contraction to the force exerted.

longer times, see Figure 5.11, which shows that 50% of maximum load can be held for one minute but 15–20% can be sustained for quite long periods. The reason for the very short maximum muscular effort is that the biochemical changes sustaining cross-bridging utilize local constituents, which can not be replaced due to the absence of blood flow. During strong isometric muscle contraction, the bulging of the muscle fibres compresses, and thus obstructs, the vessels. At lower muscle tensions, this effect is less marked and some blood flow occurs; at 15–20% of maximum tension the flow is thought to be unaffected (Grandjean, 1980). If, instead of continuous muscle contraction, a series of maximal, or near maximal, contractions (as occurs in the therapeutic application of weight resistance using, say, the 10 RM), then a similar relationship is found. Thus, lifting greater weights is associated with the ability to perform fewer repetitions and vice versa (Berger, 1982), e.g. the 10 RM (repetition maximum) is about 80% of the 1 RM. In all these circumstances the active muscles come to feel fatigued.

If activity is strenuous, prolonged and involves large muscle groups, there are marked systemic responses; increased heart and respiration rates, rise of body temperature and so forth. When these have been provoked for some time they also give rise to reduced muscle contractions as well as subjective feelings of fatigue. This may be called central fatigue to distinguish it from the local or peripheral fatigue, described above.

The mechanisms of neither of these types of fatigue are fully elucidated. From what has been said already, local fatigue is evidently not due to diminished motor neurone activity. Various metabolic changes, e.g. the increased acidity and accumulation of lactic acid, have often been considered as the important factor, but it is not a simple matter. More recent research implicates effects on potassium ion fluxes. Similarly, the causes of central fatigue are equally uncertain and include neural input, the increased body temperature, the systemic acidosis, and a rise in potassium ions. For a full and valuable discussion of these factors see Holder-Powell and Jones, 1990. In many normal activities, both types of fatigue occur but the balance between them is uncertain. In general, it is believed that the more complex the activity the more the central changes are dominant (Holder-Powell and Jones, 1990). It should be noted that the word 'fatigue' is used in many contexts with differing connotations. Psychological or mental fatigue is associated with prolonged mental activity and sleep deprivation, and is linked to boredom. To achieve an increase in muscle strength or endurance it is necessary to exercise the muscle to the point of fatigue. Advice is frequently proffered on the lines that activity should not be unduly fatiguing, although no evidence or reasons are provided.

ASSESSMENT OF MUSCLE STRENGTH

From a clinical point of view it is of great importance to be able to quantify muscle strength. This is actually done by using some method of assessing the turning force – torque – on body segments, and inferring the muscle, or muscle group, force from that. It will be, of course, proportional. There are several methods in use to measure the force exerted by the limb segment:

1. Estimating on the basis of a simple, 6-point grading system known as the Oxford scale in which:
   No evident muscle contraction = 0;
   A flicker of contraction = 1;
   A movement of the segment without outside resistance (i.e. not against the force of gravity) = 2;
   A movement of the segment against gravity = 3;
   A movement of the segment against gravity as well as some external resistance = 4;
   Normal force = 5.
2. Manual muscle testing in which the tester makes a judgement as a percentage of the normal, often in comparison with the opposite side. Being highly subjective it is notably unreliable.
3. Lifting known weights at a fixed rate in a repeatable situation. This is widely known and used to find the 10 RM and 1 RM (de Lorme and Watkins, 1957) The '1 repetition maximum' (in spite of being a contradiction in terms!) is used to denote a single maximum strength concentric contraction. Provided the technique of application is carefully standardized, with weights applied in the same position on the limb segment, the same range of motion used and so forth, then the method has reasonable reliability. Apart from fixing the weight directly to the limb, as in Figures 5.4 and 5.6, the load can be applied via lever and pulley systems, with the weights being lifted up a fixed channel. These machines are

widely used for muscle training in rehabilitation and fitness centres (the 'Multigym' for example), and dictate the position and range of motion of the body segment involved. The leverage system and friction between the moving parts means that the force exerted will not be the same as the weights applied, but will be consistent and hence provide a repeatable test. Such systems are limited to particular movements and usually to the larger muscle groups.

4. Tension-measuring devices in which the stretching out of some form of spring is used. At its simplest a spring balance can be attached (by canvas sling or other convenient method) to the body segment while the other end is fixed or held in a position to resist the contraction of a particular muscle group. This is clinically convenient and simple, and considered to be reliable provided care is taken to ensure consistent positioning. It can only measure isometric contractions. Various more specific devices are also found, which work on the same principle, for example, the cable tensiometer or isometric dynamometer. Likewise, there are a number of spring-resisted devices for single actions, such as a grip dynamometer. (The term 'dynamometer' refers to any instrument for measuring force, so all these described are dynamometers.)

5. Pressure-measuring devices are also used. The instrument is hand held against the skin and the subject attempts movement, which is resisted by the tester through the device which displays the pressure measured by a piezo-electric or other displacement transducer. With appropriate care in positioning and application technique, these systems have been shown to give reliable and repeatable results (Hyde *et al.*, 1983). Such devices are sometimes called myometers. The force plate considered in Chapter 3 measures force in the same way. Measuring air pressure has also been used, a simple rubber bulb being compressed in the hand as a grip dynamometer, for example. This has also been done with the folded cuff of an ordinary mercury column sphygmomanometer for measuring weak movements.

6. Isokinetic dynamometers are complex electromechanical devices, which control the velocity and range of limb segment motion, at the same time measuring the force exerted at a constant angular velocity. Thus, they are able to display the forces generated isotonically at different fixed velocities, as well as isometrically at any predetermined joint angle. Some modern devices are also able to assess eccentric contraction. See Jones and Barker (1995, Chapter 11) or Dvir (1995) for a description and discussion of the application of this device. A good deal of useful information can be recorded and analysed by an appropriate computer program linked to the machine. It is considered to give reasonably replicable results but there are several sources of inaccuracy (Mayhew and Rothstein, 1985).

7. A different approach, not involving the torque on the limb segment, is the use of electromyography, which measures the electrical signals – spike potentials – generated by muscle contraction. The signals are collected, summated and stored electrically from surface or intramuscular electrodes, and bear an approximate relationship to the degree of neuromuscular activity and hence muscle contraction. This is approximate because motor

unit activity will not necessarily all be detected (see *Electrotherapy Explained*, 2nd edition, Chapter 5). This is the only direct method of assessment but it should be noted that it is an assessment of muscle activity, not muscle force and is inevitably quantitatively somewhat unreliable.

In all these methods of testing, the results are dependent on the subject making a maximum voluntary effort to achieve the maximum possible muscle contraction. While a co-operative, healthy and well motivated young adult subject (on whom most of the tests of repeatability have been conducted) seems able to repeat the same maximum voluntary contraction force fairly well, they are by no means perfectly consistent. It is usually recommended that the tester should verbally encourage the subject to make a maximum effort. Although there is some support for the effectiveness of this approach (Peacock *et al.*, 1981), there is other contradictory evidence. Certainly, verbal encouragement is an effective way of increasing muscular endurance, shown in a particularly valuable and well conducted study by Bickers (1993). However, it is not certain that muscle force is affected in the same way. The actual force generated and measured by any of these methods is, of course, critically dependent on the technique adopted. Thus, the site at which the resistance of the measuring device is applied is important, as has been explained earlier. For example, placing the myometer on the limb segment closer to the joint being moved will give a higher reading. For comparable readings, strict attention to repeating the identical technique in terms of whole body and limb segment position, angle of joint or range of motion, site of fixation of the apparatus, and exhortation, are essential. Force changes in the same subject are usually the measure of interest, an increase in strength due to exercise therapy or a decrease due to progressive disease, for example. There will be very large differences between subjects and it may also be of interest to see how individuals compare with the 'normal' in terms of muscle force. There is a very good positive correlation between muscle strength and body weight (for adults, at least), as would be expected. For the quadriceps, one study found the correlation to be 0.92 (Edwards *et al.*, 1977). Thus, comparisons can be made between individuals of similar weight while allowing for the numerous other variables such as age (considered in Chapter 4) and customary exercise.

It has already been noted that muscle force is related to cross-sectional area so that measurements of limb circumference might also be used to assess muscle strength. This is difficult to do accurately, so that small changes in muscle cross-section are indetectable in the large errors that occur. The use of ultrasonic reflections to develop a cross-sectional picture with the aid of computer analysis has given much greater accuracy (Young and Hughes, 1982; Howe and Oldham, 1995). Furthermore, quite large changes in muscle strength are able to occur without corresponding changes in muscle tissue volume. Thus, gains in muscle strength occur as a result of exercise before any muscle hypertrophy occurs and, furthermore, training one set of limb muscles can lead to increased strength in the same muscles of the contralateral limb. These effects are due to changes in the central nervous system, known as neural adaptation. They have been recognized as changes in the EMG. It seems that when a muscle training programme is undertaken, the initial strength gain is principally due to neural adaptation as is also the 'cross-training' effect, while subsequent strength gains are due to both neural adaptation and hypertrophy, the latter becoming dominant after about four weeks (Moritani, 1993).

Thus, in summary, it seems that human voluntary muscle strength depends on:

1. The quantity of muscle tissue, i.e. cross-sectional area;
2. The quality of the muscle tissue, i.e. the fibre type;
3. The extent and type of neural activation of the muscle.

These can all be altered by training. The torque generated by particular limb segments depends on the way in which the muscle contracts, the velocity of contraction and the initial muscle length and architecture. The unalterable mechanical factors discussed in this chapter, the position of muscle attachments and the angle of muscle pull, also determine the torque.

6. Friction, viscosity and joint movement

As explained in Chapter 2, in terms of Newton's third law, a body resting on a surface not only exerts a downward force but experiences an equal upward acting force: the reaction force. Thus, the surfaces are pressed together. However, any force applied parallel to the surfaces is also opposed by a force that acts to try to prevent sliding of one surface on another. This force is called *friction* and it arises whenever one body moves, or tries to move, over the surface of another. It is universal and hence taken for granted, but it is of the utmost importance. The ability to walk or travel in any vehicle, securing any structure with nails or screws, and the clinging together of fibres to allow the formation of woven or knitted clothes, all depend on friction.

The simple situation, illustrated in Figure 6.1, shows the forces on an object resting on a surface, say a book on a table. If the table is tilted up as in Figure 6.1b, then the force pressing the surfaces together is diminished and some part of the downward force acts against the frictional force. At a sufficient angle, the object will slide on the surface; the force of static friction has been overcome. At what angle this will occur depends only on the nature of the two surfaces and is the ratio of the frictional force to the reaction force. This ratio is constant for a given pair of surfaces and is the *coefficient of static friction* (μ). Values for μ vary with the materials and

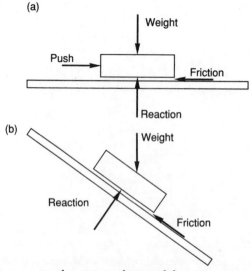

Fig. 6.1 Diagrams to show static frictional force.

nature (roughness) of the surfaces involved and are very different if a fluid – a lubricant – is placed between them. Thus, friction depends only on the nature of the surfaces and the force pressing them together. Some examples are listed in Table 6.1; note that this refers to static friction in which no motion occurs between the surfaces but, of course, when there is motion, friction is still present and is called kinetic friction. Energy has to be used to overcome this force. The coefficient of kinetic friction (also known as dynamic or sliding friction) is generally less than that of static friction (also called limiting friction) for any given pair of surfaces. It is a common experience that once the sliding of surfaces starts (the book on the tilted table of Figure 6.1 or a foot on a muddy slope), it tends to continue for this reason. Kinetic friction differs in other ways. It depends on the speed of movement between the surfaces and it uses energy, which frequently appears as heat and sound. Further, it tends to modify the involved surfaces by wear. Lubricants are applied, as discussed below, to modify these effects. Some examples are given in Table 6.2. A third kind of friction is sometimes described as rolling friction. This is the resistance of a wheel or roller rotating on a flat surface, such as a car tyre on a road. There is no sliding of one surface on another but there is regular distortion of both wheel and surface, which causes heating of both, thus wasting mechanical energy. Rolling friction is typically much less than dynamic friction.

Table 6.1 Examples of the coefficient of static friction for some pairs of materials

Materials	*Coefficient of static friction (μ)*
Surfaces of healthy synovial joint	0.002–0.008
Lubricated steel on steel	0.01–0.1
Waxed wood on snow	0.04–0.14
Ice on ice	0.05–0.15
Metal on polished wood	0.1
Aluminium on skin of knuckles	0.3
Polished wood on wood	0.35
Non-lubricated steel on steel	0.15–0.6
Rubber on smooth tile	0.3–0.4
Dry wood on dry wood	0.25–0.5
Wood on stone	0.6
Leather on wood	0.62
Rubber on wood	0.7
Skin of soles of feet on wood	0.8
Skin of fingertips on aluminium	1.0
Rubber on concrete	1.2

These are only examples and considerable variation would occur depending on the exact nature of the surfaces involved.

Table 6.2 Examples of the coefficient of kinetic or sliding friction for some pairs of materials

Materials	Coefficient of kinetic friction
Normal hip joint	0.002
Steel on ice	0.01
Cobalt-chromium on polyethylene	0.08
Cobalt-chromium on cobalt-chromium	0.12
Leather on wood	0.4
Rubber on concrete	0.7

From Dumbleton and Black, 1981.

It is helpful to consider what happens between two surfaces at a microscopic level. Since no practical surface can be perfectly flat, the tiny irregularities (asperities) that make up each surface press on to the other surface only at their tips (see Fig. 6.2). The real area of contact is thus much smaller than the apparent area. The more firmly the surfaces are compressed, the more the asperities mutually engage and the larger the area of real contact and the sliding of one surface on another therefore becomes more difficult, i.e. friction is greater. This explains several features of friction: the fact that smoother surfaces seem to correlate approximately with low friction and that friction is independent of apparent surface contact area. It also explains the way in which lubricants can work; they separate the surfaces, keeping the asperities apart so that movement now occurs between the lubricant molecules.

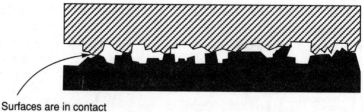

Surfaces are in contact
only at the asperities

Fig. 6.2 Enlarged cross-section of two surfaces in contact.

Table 6.1 illustrates a very large range of friction coefficients, from the quite astonishingly small frictional forces in synovial joints, considered further below, to the large forces between the rubber, say, of a tyre, and concrete. It is striking how much less friction occurs in synovial joints than in even well engineered metal-on-metal joints. Skiers and skaters are familiar with the low friction between smooth waxed skis and snow and the steel of skates with ice (Table 6.2). In both cases, the movement over the surface leads to some melting, providing water as a lubricant. In many circumstances, high frictional forces are needed, such as between the foot and the ground, or the rubber tyre and the road. In a physiotherapeutic context, the rubber ferrule of a crutch or stick should not be able to slide easily over the surface on which it is used. Table 6.1 shows the greater coefficient of friction between rubber and concrete compared with rubber on smooth tile (which may be even less if the tile is wet, the water acting as a lubricant). In this connection, it may be noted that, for maximum friction, footwear is adapted for the surface on which it is to be used. Thus, on soft surfaces such as mud or snow, projections are deliberately provided to 'dig in' and prevent sliding, as in studs on football boots, crampons, hob-nailed boots for example. On surfaces that do not deform, such as smooth stone, this is not effective and the low coefficient of friction between the smooth nail heads and the stone makes these unsafe footwear in this situation. Human skin shows frictional properties appropriate to its function. Thus, the skin of the foot has a coefficient of friction of around 0.8 on wooden boards. Similarly, the skin of the palm of the hand has a much higher coefficient of friction than that of the dorsum, the fingertips, being about 1 on aluminium (Table 6.1; Alexander, 1992). Clearly, the ridged and slightly wrinkled surface of the plantar and palmar skin surfaces are adapted to gripping the surface to which they are applied. Other parts of the skin, especially when dry and smooth, exhibit very much lower friction. Physiotherapists applying the steel or aluminium head of an ultrasonic applicator, even with a layer of fluid couplant, may notice these differences when moving over palmar, plantar and other surfaces. Slight sweating of the palms and soles seems to increase friction, perhaps because it removes oils on the surface such as naturally produced sebum.

Walking in shoes with leather, rubber or plastic composite material as the undersurface on polished, carpeted or other flooring is safe, as there is usually good frictional resistance. This may not be so with some polishes or with water or other lubricants on the floor. It has been found that the horizontal component of heel strike and toe off during normal walking is about 15–20% of body weight (Williams and Lissner, 1962), which would suggest that the coefficient of static friction between the surfaces should be at least 0.2. However, the actual force at both heel strike and toe off will be greater than the body weight, so this is an overestimate.

Lubrication to reduce friction has been widely studied – known as tribology (from the Greek 'tribos' meaning rubbing) – mainly for the movement of one metal part on another in engineering. Oils, greases and graphite are widely used. The central problem is to maintain a layer of lubricant between the moving surfaces. *Hydrodynamic lubrication* achieves this because when one part moves continuously relative to another, such as a rotating shaft in a fixed bearing, it drags oil with it, continually replenishing the layer of oil between the surfaces. In many parts of a reciprocating engine there is a cyclical variation of pressure between the surfaces. At high pressure, the oil is squeezed but not completely ejected from the space between the surfaces before the pressure is reduced allowing the oil film to thicken again. This is known as *squeeze film lubrication*. Even when all the oil is removed from metal-bearing surfaces there still remain some molecules attached to the surfaces that help to maintain separation and provide what is called *boundary lubrication*. All these forms of lubrication depend to some extent on the viscosity and properties of adherence and elasticity of the lubricant. In many bearings, it is possible to have all these forms of lubrication at different times, i.e. *mixed lubrication*. In some circumstances the lubricant is forced between the surfaces by external pressure — the oil is pumped into the bearing — this is *hydrostatic lubrication*.

It may be wondered how biological joints have such exceptionally low friction. The articular cartilage forms the bearing surfaces and the synovial fluid is the lubricant contained by the joint capsule lined with synovial membrane. It is considered that some mixed lubrication occurs, notably squeeze film lubrication (because regularly varying, oscillating pressure takes place in many cyclical activities such as walking), together with boundary lubrication. However, it seems there are different features that allow joints to move with such low friction. These are mainly due to the fact that articular cartilage is not rigid and solid but elastic and rather porous, as described in Chapter 2. Thus, the surfaces deform slightly under pressure, giving a more evenly matched pair of surfaces and, importantly, allowing fluid to be squeezed slowly in and out of the cartilage. Because the synovial fluid is trapped between the irregularities on the surface of the cartilage it maintains a fluid layer. In spite of its smooth, glassy appearance, articular cartilage is actually quite irregular at microscopic level. This is called *weeping lubrication*. It can be partly simulated by firmly wiping a water-filled sponge on a smooth metal or enamel surface. The structure of articular cartilage was discussed in Chapter 2 and it will be recalled that it consists mainly of water ($\approx 75\%$) contained in a skeleton of collagen with some (5%) special proteoglycan molecules. These draw water into the cartilage, which is prevented from swelling by the collagen skeleton. Thus, the cartilage is a wet rubbery material whose surface will weep when it is compressed. When cartilage is pressed on at first, the water is driven slowly to parts that are under less pressure but this becomes more difficult as the fluid content falls. Synovial fluid contains proteins and hyaluronic acid, which make it viscous. The water can be squeezed out through the cartilage, but the larger hyaluronic and protein molecules cannot. Therefore the layer of lubricating molecules between the cartilage surfaces becomes more concentrated and hence more viscous. It can be seen that the nature of the lubricant is being adjusted to suit the load conditions of the joint. The concept is called *boosted lubrication* and has no evident parallel in engineering joints. While these ideas go some way to account for the efficiency of biological joints there is still a good deal of uncertainty, particularly with regard to the importance of each mechanism in different joint-loading conditions. While great progress has been made with artificial replacement hip joints it can be seen in Table 6.2

that they have much greater kinetic friction than natural joints.

It is hardly surprising that much effort is put into trying to reduce friction in machinery of all kinds since it is wasteful of energy. It has been suggested that about 20% of the energy used in a modern car is lost as friction in the moving parts. Not only does the friction waste energy it also causes heat, which has to be dissipated, and wear on the surfaces, which have to be replaced.

There are many physiotherapeutic situations in which frictional forces are modified by altering the surface pressure or the lubricant. The ultrasound couplant noted above not only provides a means of passing ultrasonic energy to the tissues but also allows relatively friction-free motion of the treatment head on the skin surface. Similarly, to allow smooth movements of skin on skin, as in the application of therapeutic massage, powder or oil is used as a lubricant. The importance of a suitable high frictional force between the foot and the ground has already been considered. It is quite a simple matter to find the approximate coefficient of friction between any particular shoe and flooring. The shoe is loaded with an appropriate known weight and a hand-held spring balance is attached. This is then pulled along the floor surface by the spring balance, which is kept parallel to the floor. Readings are taken just before the shoe moves and during steady motion (to give values for static and kinetic friction respectively). Several readings with different weights may be taken. The brakes on wheelchairs and bed casters depend on adequate friction between the moving surface and the brake pad. The coefficient of friction for a brake-shoe on a brake-drum is usually around 1.2. Many pieces of apparatus for providing resistance to muscular exercise use friction to absorb the energy, such as a static bicycle using either a belt on a revolving drum or air resistance. The static frictional forces between shoes and flooring surfaces are often quite large but, as can be seen from Table 6.2, once movement occurs, the kinetic friction or sliding friction is much lower; compare the figures for leather on wood, and rubber on concrete, for example. Lubricants such as oil or water will markedly lower both frictional forces; sliding friction between wet rubber and wet concrete is about 0.5.

It has been suggested that only the gross irregularities of a surface dictate the frictional forces, but this is too simple. There will be secondary adherence of atoms and molecules to one another with varying forces depending on their nature, as well as electrical interactions, which may cause attraction between the surfaces. Some engineering lubricants act by binding to, and thus modifying, the bearing surfaces.

VISCOSITY

It was noted above that lubricants exhibit viscosity. This is the property of a fluid that enables it to resist flowing when shear stresses are applied to it. Thus, fluids with a high viscosity are sticky and flow slowly like treacle

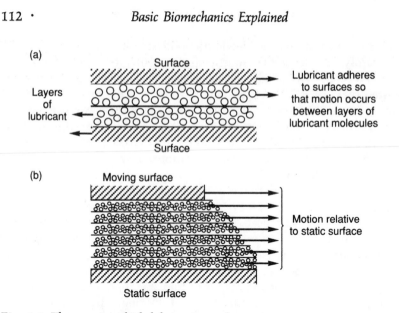

Fig. 6.3 The way in which lubricants work.

or thick oil. Where a fluid moves over a rigid surface, as happens in lubricated bearings, the layer of fluid in contact with the surface tends to remain stationary while the adjacent layer of molecules moves slowly over it, and the next layer over that one and so on. Thus the motion is spread over several layers of molecules, the ones more distant from the surface moving faster with respect to the surface (see Fig. 6.3). Viscous forces act to resist the different rates of motion of different layers. The same occurs whatever the motion of the fluid, so that viscosity is a measure of the ease with which the fluid molecules move with respect to one another. It is like kinetic friction between surfaces, except that it acts through the bulk of the fluid. If a fluid is moved over a rigid surface, or vice versa, it is found that the resistance to fluid motion is directly proportional to the speed of movement, the area of contact, viscosity, and inversely proportional to fluid thickness. The viscosity, η, is a constant that is characteristic of a particular fluid. It is a measure of how much force is needed to move one part of the fluid over another, measured in newton seconds per square metre (Ns m^{-2}). These SI units are poiseuilles or pascal seconds (in the cgs system it is called a poise; 1 poiseuille = 10 poise). For many fluids, viscosity is constant — called newtonian fluids — but in others it varies with greater shearing force, rising in some, called dilutants, and diminishing with time in others, called thixotropic liquids.

Since viscosity depends on the ease with which molecules move with respect to one another, it would be expected that a temperature rise would lead to reduced viscosity in liquids; this is what occurs. Hence, viscosities are given for a particular temperature. In gases, the reverse occurs in that viscosity increases with temperature. (For a simple account of the behaviour of materials with changes in temperature see *Physical Principles Explained*.) Some examples are given in Table 6.3. This table also demonstrates that viscosity is unrelated to density; mercury is less viscid but much more dense than glycerine, and water more dense than oil but less viscid. A central difference between viscous and frictional forces is that viscosity only occurs during motion, while friction can be found both when surfaces are moving on one another and when they are not, i.e. static friction.

Table 6.3 Values of viscosity (η) in some fluids

Fluid	Temperature (°C)	Viscosity (Poiseuilles (Ns m^{-2}))
Liquids		
Water	20	1.0×10^{-3}
Water	37	6.91×10^{-4}
Water	100	2.82×10^{-4}
Alcohol	20	1.2×10^{-3}
Olive oil	20	8.4×10^{-2}
Mercury	20	1.55×10^{-3}
Mercury	100	1.2×10^{-3}
Glycerine	20	1.5
Light machine oil	38	3.4×10^{-2}
Gases		
Air	0	1.71×10^{-5}
Air	18	1.82×10^{-5}
Air	40	1.9×10^{-5}
Hydrogen	20	8.8×10^{-6}
Water vapour	100	1.25×10^{-5}

VISCOELASTICITY

Elastic behaviour was considered in Chapter 2; some tissues of the body have properties of both elasticity and viscosity. Thus, slow deformation of the tissue occurs elastically but rapid deformation is strongly resisted because of viscous resistance; viscosity will be a greater resistance at higher velocities. Synovial fluid behaves in this way. A model to gain insight into viscoelasticity can be imagined replacing the cross-bridging representation of Figure 4.6 with something that represents viscous resistance – a piston moving in a tin of treacle provides an appropriate mental image – so that parallel and series elastic elements act with a viscous element.

RESISTANCE TO MOVEMENT OF NORMAL SYNOVIAL JOINTS

In the preceding two chapters, the ways in which muscle can act on joints was considered and the weight of the segments being measured – the effect of gravity on the mass of the parts – was noted as an external force resisting motion. Other external forces, lifted weights, manual resistance etc. were also noted. What of the 'internal' forces that resist and restrict joint movement? Clearly, they are quite significant because, if a totally relaxed limb is allowed to swing freely, it comes to rest after four or five swings. In pathological conditions, such as arthritis, the patient complains of stiffness, which is a subjective feeling of difficulty in moving joints.

First, inertia of the body part being moved will provide resistance to motion. This depends on mass and acceleration, as described in Chapter 1. Thus, a large body segment, such as the leg, will need more force to start it moving than a small one, such as a finger. Secondly, all the tissues are distorted in some way, by being stretched, compressed etc. and resist this change elastically, as described in Chapter 2. The elastic resistance increases with the displacement mainly in a non-linear manner (see Fig. 2.11). Thus, it is found that elastic resistance increases greatly and is a major limiting force at the extremes of joint range. It is this force that ultimately limits joint motion and is contributed to by many tissues, ligaments, skin, etc. In living joints, as the stretch increases, so muscle contraction occurs to prevent tissue damage.

Thirdly, during joint motion, the movement is resisted by the viscosity of the tissues. This, as explained, will be at its maximum during the most rapid motion; hence, in normal joint movement, it will be greatest in the middle of the range. It will be more significant during fast motion than when the joint is moved slowly. It is not only the tissues about the joint that are involved but also those at a considerable distance that are affected by the movement of a joint, such as a muscle acting on a long tendon and the tendon itself perhaps moving in a synovial sheath.

Fourthly, the movement of articular cartilage on cartilage or other tissue is resisted by friction. Friction is dependent on the load on the joint: the force pressing the surfaces together. While the weight-bearing joints of the lower limbs normally bear the greatest compressive forces, all joint surfaces are compressed by muscle action to achieve stability.

The relative contribution of each of these resistive forces has been investigated under various circumstances and considerable variation has been found. In the fingers, elastic resistance was found to be by far the greatest (90%), while viscosity contributed 9% and friction a negligible 1%. Similar relationships were found for the knee but viscosity and friction made larger contributions. As might be expected, inertial resistance was negligible in the finger but significant in the knee (Wright, 1973). Marked variations occur between subjects and joints, and, from time to time, even in the same joint. In general, friction appears to make only a minor contribution to resisting motion in healthy joints, the major component being the elastic resistance of the surrounding tissues.

Two further points must be made in connection with time. If the joint is held in an extreme position, the force needed to hold it there diminishes with time. Secondly, in any part of the range of movement, viscoelastic effects, as noted above, may mean that full elastic recovery does not occur. Synovial fluid is a viscoelastic substance, so initial rapid changes tend to be resisted elastically, but it subsequently behaves as a viscous material giving a lower constant resistance to motion. (It is this quality of the mucus exuded by the 'foot' of limpets, slugs and snails that enables them to move without losing contact with the surface (Alexander, 1992).)

In summary, then, normal joint motion is resisted by internal forces of:

elasticity, which depends on joint displacement;
viscosity, which depends on joint velocity;
friction, which depends on joint loading;
inertia, which depends on tissue mass.

For small joints that are moving small segments, elasticity is much the most important component. For larger, more heavily loaded joints, the other forces become more significant.

There are many physiological circumstances that affect the resistance to movement or 'stiffness' of normal joints. As might be expected, there is, on average, some increased stiffness of joints with age. There is apparently a very wide scatter, with some elderly people being very little different from young adults (Beighton *et al.*, 1983). A survey on male knees found that men in their sixties were, on average, some 23.2% stiffer than those in their twenties; again a wide scatter of readings was found (Wright, 1973). The joints in females tend to be less stiff than those of males. One explanation for this is the fact that joints are smaller on average. It has also been suggested (Beighton *et al.*, 1983) that there is a variation among races, Africans and, to a lesser extent, Indians being more mobile than Europeans. One circumstance in which subjective stiffness is experienced in the joints of healthy subjects is that of local cooling. If the hand is cooled to a skin temperature of 18°C, objective measurement has shown an increased resistance to motion of some 10–20%. Superficial and deep tissue heating (with shortwave diathermy) has been shown to produce the reverse effect. This is to be expected in view of the influence of temperature on viscosity.

The difference in joint mobility with age, as noted above, did not consider children, whose joint mobility is very great indeed. In fact, mobility appears to diminish rapidly with age to adulthood and then more slowly (Beighton *et al.*, 1983).

Joint mobility due to disease can be reduced, both as a loss of the normal range of motion and as subjective stiffness, or it can be increased. The former is common and familiar due to tissue trauma or joint disease, while the latter, called the hypermobility syndrome, is relatively rare. Hypermobility may be due to genetic disorders of connective tissue such as the Ehlers–Danlos or Marfan syndromes, or simply an extreme of the normal variation in joint mobility. Excessively mobile joints appear to predispose to degenerative joint disorders. The causes of hypermobility, or hyperlaxity, are complex but are believed to be a deficiency of connective tissue, either due to loss of the normal 'crimp' of the collagen fibres (see Chapter 2) or some biochemical abnormality, or both. Loss of mobility is often due to increased quantities of connective tissue, i.e. abnormal amounts of scarring, in places where it restricts tissue movement (adhesions).

AIR RESISTANCE

In considering the forces, both external and internal, that act to resist body or body segment movement, one force that has not been considered so far is the resistance of the medium through which the body moves. The effects of water on body motion are discussed in Chapter 7 and are very significant, but air resistance is so small at normal rates of motion that it is usually ignored. This resistance is due to the viscosity of air and acts in the way just described; that is, the molecules on the body surface tend to adhere to the skin and move with respect to the air molecules in the next layer. Because the viscosity of air is so low (see Table 6.3), the resistance at the usual everyday velocities of body movement is negligible. However, as noted already, it is critically dependent on velocity so that in activities like skiing, skating or cycling, in which the body moves at quite high velocities, it becomes important. It will be noted that downhill skiers, racing skaters and cyclists all adopt special postures to minimize air resistance. (While inept amateur skiers and skaters may be too distracted while adopting special and often undignified postures to notice air resistance, most have experienced the difficulty of cycling into the wind!) Even at the relatively low velocities of sprinters, air resistance is a significant factor as evidenced by the effect on sprint records at altitudes with lower air density. It may be seen that sprinting is performed with rapid forward movement of a markedly bent knee, as opposed to endurance running in which the limb remains relatively straight. This is done to 'shorten' the limb so that it has less inertia on rapid forward movement but it also makes it have less resistance to moving through air.

Consider a sky-diver falling through the air under the acceleration due to gravity of a constant $9.81\,m\,s^{-2}$. As the falling speed increases so does the 'drag' or friction due to the air. This is illustrated in Figure 6.4a in which the force due to drag is plotted against the velocity. There comes a point at which the resistance due to drag is equal to the downward driving force of gravity when the velocity is at maximum (called the terminal velocity). This velocity then remains constant and is about $60\,m\,s^{-1}$. The terminal velocity can, of course, be reduced with increased drag resistance by opening a parachute, for example, which gives a terminal velocity in the region of 7 ms⁻¹ (Fig. 6.4b). In the activities considered above, in which the body is propelled horizontally by muscular

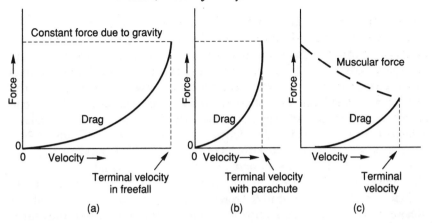

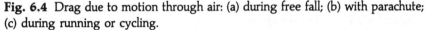

Fig. 6.4 Drag due to motion through air: (a) during free fall; (b) with parachute; (c) during running or cycling.

activity, cycling, skating, etc., the same factors apply but the driving force is no longer constant. In general, the faster the muscles are made to contract the less force they can generate, as noted in Chapter 4. Thus, as the body is propelled more rapidly by more rapidly moving limbs, so the maximum force that can be generated becomes less; Figure 6.4c illustrates this. Air resistance for athletes running at, say, $6\,\mathrm{m\,s^{-1}}$ is quite significant for running races. It may be thought that a circular track would eliminate the advantage of a tail wind with the disadvantage of the ensuing head wind, but this is not quite the case because the athlete spends relatively longer slowed by the head wind than aided by the tail wind.

The air resistance to motion of rapidly revolving vanes is used in therapeutic exercise devices such as rowing machines and static bicycles, as mentioned above.

THERAPEUTIC PASSIVE MOVEMENT

Moving synovial joints by an outside force, usually manually, has been used therapeutically for many years. It is usual to describe manually or mechanically produced rhythmical motion within the normal available joint range as relaxed passive movements. If the joint motion can be produced only actively in the presence of some outside resistance, such as rotation of the metacarpals around a grasped ball or the distraction of a joint, it is called an accessory movement. Relaxed passive movements are utilized therapeutically in circumstances in which normal active motion is temporarily not possible or not desirable; they serve to maintain the normal joint range and muscle length. The deleterious effects of prolonged joint immobilization are well recognized.

While relaxed passive movements have been manually applied therapeutically from antiquity, their continuous application by mechanical means is relatively recent. Devices that will move the limb segments through a preset range at a fixed rate for several hours each day are available in many hospitals. Some evidence for the value of such continuous passive movement has been provided. A comparison between total knee arthroplasty patients given a standardized exercise programme and those additionally receiving continuous passive movement found that the latter had an improved range of motion, appeared to have lower pain levels and left hospital earlier (Harms and Engstrom, 1991). Similarly, evidence for its value in ankle fractures has been presented (Davies, 1991). Coutts *et al.* (1989) consider that continuous passive movement allows knee flexion to be achieved and maintained with greater ease and less discomfort for the patient in the short term. It is, therefore, a useful adjunct in the postoperative treatment of various joint conditions. Research (on animals) has suggested that continuous passive movement can encourage the healing and regeneration of articular-type cartilage. Clinical studies have provided some support for the belief that pain and the risk of deep vein thrombosis are both reduced with continuous passive movement therapy, which does not appear to delay wound healing. However, a major justification for its use, and indeed for the use of manually applied relaxed passive movements, seems to be a recognition of the value of moderate joint motion.

JOINT MEASUREMENT

The measurement of the position and range of motion of joints is of central importance in the clinical situation. A knowledge of the changes that occur over time is essential to providing proper therapy and for research. There are two aspects:

1. Measuring static joint position, thus describing a fixed deformity or the possible range of free joint motion: this is the simplest, most useful approach and will be considered first;
2. Measuring and recording the motion, a dynamic measurement, during activity: this provides not only the available range of motion but also can be used to assess the amount of motion over a particular time.

Static joint measurement can be carried out by simple estimation, but better reliability is achieved with the use of some angle-measuring device, known as a goniometer (Low, 1976a), of which there are numerous types. The universal goniometer has a 360° scale with two long arms, one pivoted at the centre to allow free movement. Pendulum or bubble goniometers are used to relate the angle of the body segment to the vertical. In some parts of the body, for example the spine or the fingers, the angles between the segments may be more conveniently measured with a malleable metal strip or wire. A permanent record is made by drawing around the strip on paper. A similar permanent record can be made for some movements by drawing around the part on a sheet of paper, e.g. abduction of the fingers. A photocopier can be used in a similar way for the fingers and wrists (Metcalf and Yeabel, 1972). Photography is also used but is technically difficult. Radiography of the part may also provide information but, of course, would not be used repetitively due to the risk of tissue damage. Linear measurement, made with a tape measure or ruler, may be used to determine the range of motion of a joint or series of joints, e.g. side flexion of the lumbar spine. Many special devices and methods have been described for particular joints, each having advantages of simplicity or accuracy, for example, large collar-type goniometers to measure rotation in the cervical spine. A brief account of several of these can be found in Low, 1976b. Of all these different approaches, goniometry with a universal goniometer is by far the most widely used and recommended because of its simplicity (Gajdosik and Bohannon, 1987). There are several descriptions of the techniques (e.g. Norkin and White, 1985; American Academy of Orthopedic Surgeons, 1965).

Technique of goniometry

It is necessary to determine precisely how the joint position being measured is to be maintained, either actively or passively. If actively, it is usual to instruct the patient to move as far as possible within the limits of pain; if passively, the investigator applies the force. In both cases it is important that the same force is repeated at subsequent measurements to ensure repeatability. The position of the patient and the posture of both proximal and distal joints must be standardized and repeated at subsequent measurements. The axis of the goniometer must be placed over the axis of the joint. Since no joint motion is exactly uniaxial, as noted above, this is inevitably an approximation. In hinge-type movements, the bony attachment of the collateral ligament provides a guide, e.g. the epicondyles of the humerus and femur, the tips of the malleoli, and the styloid process of the radius and ulna. The arms of the goniometer are applied parallel to the mid-line of the limb segment. Sometimes it is more convenient to apply the arms of the goniometer to the surface of the limb segment rather than the mid-line. The most important aspect of the technique is that it must be repeated as exactly as possible for each measurement in order to achieve reliability.

Reliability of goniometric measurement

The technique used and its repeatability is of prime importance in achieving reliable measurements (Nicol, 1989). It has been suggested (Hellebrandt et al., 1949) that failure to align the axis of the goniometer correctly is the largest single source of error. In general, intra-tester reliability has been found to be very much greater than inter-tester reliability (Low, 1976a; Boone *et al.*, 1978). The latter recommend that, if the same observer takes all the measurements, then changes beyond 3° or 4°should be detected before a real change in range is accepted. Inter-tester measurement should be beyond 5° for the upper and 6° for the lower limb. Using the mean of several observations is considered to improve accuracy, but not all agree (e.g. Boone *et al.*, 1978). Even the rather large errors found in other studies of clinical goniometry (Low, 1976a) do not diminish the value since these are relatively small variations considering the magnitude of real changes. It has been suggested that some of the variation may be due to slight normal day to day changes in tissue tension. Real pathological limitations tend to be much larger. Several of the special measuring instruments or special techniques for particular clinical measurements, such as straight leg raising or lumbar side flexion, have been investigated with regard to their repeatability. Many of the specialist devices exhibit high levels of reliability in the hands of their protagonists. However, confirmation in a clinical setting is often lacking. In fact, investigation of some widely used clinical measurements has sometimes shown poorer reliability than expected (e.g. Rose, 1991).

An example of a linear measurement is the measurement of the height that a patient can reach up a wall as a method of assessing shoulder complex function. This is a widely used, simple assessment but subject to many sources of error. For example, the patient needs to adopt the same position and make a similar effort on each occasion. As noted earlier, the height of the patient can vary quite significantly (up to 2 cm) during the day. A way of avoiding these errors without increasing the complexity of the measurement has been suggested by recording a comparison between the two arms (Low, 1963). This method depends on having a normal arm for comparison and is, of course, a measure of total shoulder function, which does not distinguish between glenohumeral and scapular motion. Making separate scapular and glenohumeral measurements has proved to be difficult. Youdas *et al.* (1994) concluded that the reliability of measurements using a new scapulohumeral goniometer was poor. This principle of using a measured comparison with the unaffected side has application in taking many other joint measurements and also, for that matter, measurements of limb volume or muscle strength, as discussed in Chapter 5. Muscle strength, for example, has been shown to vary with the time of day, being lower in the early morning, so that measurements either have to be repeated at the same time or, more simply, a comparison is used.

A source of error in making clinical measurements lies in the way they are recorded and communicated. Angular joint measurements are often described simply in degrees, but the starting position and the angle of the starting position must be known. The method recommended by the American Academy of Orthopedic Surgeons (1965) is widely suggested. In this, all joint movement is measured from a specified zero starting position and the fully extended 'anatomical position' is taken as 0° (except that the mid-position of shoulder and forearm rotation is used). Much difficulty can be prevented by the use of 'pinmen' diagrams on record sheets to show exactly which angle has been measured. Methods such as photography or drawing around a flexible strip provide a self-evident paper record from which changes can be measured. In all cases, the exact technique used should be noted.

Dynamic joint measurement involves a measurement of the moving joint. An electrogoniometer, which is simply a variable resistor with the contacts forming the moving limb of the goniometer (see *Physical Principles Explained*), is attached to two body segments. Movement varies the position of the contact on the wire and hence the resistance of the electrogoniometer. This output can be fed into suitable recording apparatus to provide a continuous record of joint angle against time. It is like having the joint moving the volume control knob to and fro on the radio, and recording the output. Since the electrogoniometer must be electrically connected to recording apparatus and is somewhat cumbersome, it is usually used for research applications of repetitive movements such as walking (but see below).

Historically, the oldest method of recording joint motion is by photography. Making a cinefilm, which can be examined frame by frame, usually with markers to indicate exact bony point locations for analysis, has been used. Similarly, using light-reflecting markers on a completely dark subject and keeping the camera shutter open during the regular flashing of a light, results in a picture of a series of markers in succeeding positions. From this picture, both the extent and rate of angular motion can be calculated. (For cyclical activity like walking, a stroboscope matched to the cadence can be used to assess particular positions or postures.)

With the greater availability of relatively cheap video cameras and recorders these are now sometimes used in a similar way. In clinical situations, all these methods present technical problems which tend to limit their usefulness. Furthermore, analysis of the resulting pictures is difficult and time consuming. Video cameras can now be linked to computers that analyse the movements as required.

A difficulty in using the electrogoniometer described above is that of maintaining correct alignment during joint motion, since, as noted, joints do not move around a stationary axis. This problem has been ingeniously overcome by the use of a flexible steel strip fitted with strain gauges. The electrical output of the strain gauges is proportional to the angle between the ends and is unaffected by the movement of the axes of the body segments or skin movements (Nicol, 1989). The device is fixed to the skin surface and the electrical output can be fed to a hand-held display unit computerized data processing system. It is useful that such goniometers are lightweight and can be worn under clothing, with the electrical output recorded by a special small tape recorder carried by the patient. This means that functional joint motion at home can be recorded over time. Thus, not only is information provided on the ranges of motion, rates of motion and preferred postures of the joint but also on the quantity of joint motion. Such arrangements have been used for the assessment of patients' functional movements during recovery from joint replacement surgery. This flexible strip and strain gauge has been developed to measure and record motion in two, and even three, planes thus giving more information on real joint motion.

In summary, therefore, joint motion and position may be measured by:

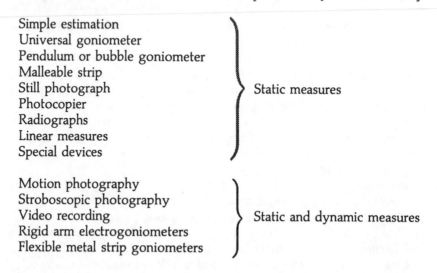

Simple estimation
Universal goniometer
Pendulum or bubble goniometer
Malleable strip
Still photograph
Photocopier
Radiographs
Linear measures
Special devices

⎫
⎬ Static measures
⎭

Motion photography
Stroboscopic photography
Video recording
Rigid arm electrogoniometers
Flexible metal strip goniometers

⎫
⎬ Static and dynamic measures
⎭

7.   *Properties of water related to hydrotherapy*

Some of the features of body movement involving fluid media have already been considered in the last chapter under lubrication and body movement through air. This chapter is intended to explain how the special properties of water influence movement and exercise. Water and similar fluids at rest will be considered and then the effect of fluid motion.

Water is a liquid with rather special properties. All liquids are characterized by having a definite volume, like solids, but, unlike solids, shape is dictated by the shape of the container. This is due to the fact that the molecules of a liquid, while being held fairly closely together, are able to move easily with respect to one another. Such movement is allowed to occur because the liquid contains sufficient energy to overcome some of the interatomic bonding forces. If some energy is removed, thus cooling the liquid, a point occurs at which solid crystals are formed, i.e. the water freezes to become solid ice. Water is unusual in that the molecules are more closely packed together at 4°C than as ice crystals. Thus, ice is less dense than water and will float. If energy is added, heating the water, it ultimately boils forming water vapour, which is a gas. This occurs because sufficient energy has been added to disrupt the bonds completely, allowing wide separation of the molecules and thus the formation of a gas. The foregoing points are discussed in *Physical Principles Explained* (pp. 155–156).

PRESSURE

In Chapter 2, the response of solids to outside force in terms of their elastic or plastic distortion was discussed; clearly, fluids (liquids, gases), being non-rigid, cannot behave in quite the same way. However, forces acting perpendicularly to the surface of fluids will tend to drive the molecules closer together. The intermolecular and interatomic forces will tend to resist any such motion (see Fig. 2.5) so that a state of pressure exists in the fluid. The concept of pressure is of great importance and is considered in more detail in Chapter 8. Pressure is defined as the force per unit area exerted perpendicularly on a surface. It is measured in newtons per square metre (pascals).

$$1 \text{ pascal} = 1 \, \text{N m}^{-2}$$

There are numerous other, often more familiar, units for measuring pressure (see Table 8.1).

There are two separate sources of pressure in a fluid: first, any outside force pressing on the fluid surface, e.g. the endocardium pressing on the blood during ventricular systole or the elastic recoil of rubber on the air in a tyre; secondly, the force of gravity on the fluid, i.e. the effect of the weight of the fluid. If the weight of the fluid itself can be neglected so that only the first circumstance applies, then the pressure in a fluid at rest is the same everywhere. This is Pascal's law. If the weight of the fluid itself is significant, then the pressure increases with depth. Of course, both sources of pressure apply in all fluids but the relative importance of the force of gravity on a fluid is critically dependent on its density.

Density is the ratio of the mass of a substance to its volume. The average density, often denoted ρ (rho) is a characteristic of any substance. Hence

$$\rho = \frac{\text{mass}}{\text{volume}}$$

Some examples of the density of common substances are shown in Table 7.1. It is evident that the density of a substance will be increased if the constituent atoms and molecules are pressed more closely together. Thus, density is greater with increased pressure and less with increased temperature when the molecules are moving further apart. The changes in solids and liquids are slight but gases are strongly temperature and pressure dependent (see Table 7.1). Densities are expressed in kilograms per cubic metre but may be more familiar as grams per cubic centimetre:

$$1\,\text{g cm}^{-3} = 10^3\,\text{kg m}^{-3}$$

The ratio of the density of a substance to that of water is called the specific gravity of that substance.

Thus, the pressure in a fluid due to its own weight depends on the density and the depth of the fluid. It will increase with depth and be greater in denser fluids. The effect is, therefore, largely negligible with gases due to their low density (see Table 7.1) and with thin fluid layers, such as the synovial fluid in a joint. On the other hand, in liquids, like water, there is a marked pressure increase with depth, which is independent of the shape of the container. The pressure in a fluid due to gravity can be shown to be the product of the force of gravity, the density and the height (depth) of the fluid. This can be expressed as:

$$\text{pressure} = g\,\rho\,h$$

where

g = acceleration due to gravity = $981\,\text{m s}^{-2}$
ρ = density of the fluid in kg m^{-3}
h = depth from surface in m

so the pressure will be in pascals or N m^{-2}.

Note that the units agree i.e.:

> metres per second per second × kg per cubic metre × metres
> = kilogram metres per second per second per square metre

or

> acceleration × density × height = force per unit area (pressure)

Table 7.1 Densities of some substances

	kg m^{-3}
Solids at 20°C	
Lead	11 300
Steel	7 700
Glass	2 600
Bone	1 600
Wood	700
Solid at 0°	
Ice	917
Liquids at 20°C	
Pure water	997
Sea water	1 025
Ethyl alcohol	791
Chloroform	1 483
Liquid at 0°C	
Pure water	1 000
Gas at 100°C	
Steam	0.596
Gas at 20°C	
Air	1.2
Gases at 0°C	
Air	1.3
Carbon dioxide	1.98
Oxygen	1.43
Nitrogen	1.25
Hydrogen	0.0899

Data in this table are from Cromer (1981); all were measured at 1.01×10^5 Pa (1 atmosphere). To find the densities in grams per cubic centimetre, which is the more familiar form for solids and liquids, it is only necessary to divide by 10^3 (i.e. 1000). Thus, the density of ice is 917 kg m^{-3} or 0.917 g cm^{-3}.

In most situations, there will be an additional force on the fluid surface, as noted above, which must be added to give the total pressure. In bodies of water, such as hydrotherapy pools, this is the atmospheric pressure. Since this has the same effect outside the water it is frequently disregarded. Pressures in body fluids, for example, are always given as the pressure in excess of the atmospheric pressure. This is technically known as the gauge pressure. Similarly, the mean air pressure in the lungs is atmospheric pressure with a small gauge pressure above during expiration and below during inspiration.

It is evident that a person standing upright in the hydrotherapy pool will have a greater pressure on his/her feet, and that this pressure will diminish progressively towards the water surface. Standing in water 1 m deep (approximately up to the anterior superior iliac spines on a 1.8 m man) would give a gauge pressure at the feet of:

$$9.81\,\mathrm{m\,s^{-2}}\ 1000\,\mathrm{kg\,m^{-3}} \times 1\,\mathrm{m} = 9810\,\mathrm{Pa}$$

In water 1.25 m deep (up to the xiphisternum on a 1.8 m man) the gauge pressure at the feet would be 12 262.5 Pa and in water 1.5 m deep (to shoulder level) it would be 14 715 Pa.

Thus, for every centimetre increase in depth, the pressure at the feet rises 98.1 Pa or about 0.75 mm Hg (see Table 8.1), which gives a pressure gradient on a subject standing or sitting up to their neck in water (see Fig. 7.1). This has quite marked effects on the cardiovascular system in that about 0.7 litre of blood normally pooled in the lower limbs is redistributed to the cardiovascular space, leading to increased cardiac output. This provokes several other physiological responses including diuresis and increased sodium excretion (Hall *et al.*, 1990). The pressure gradient will oppose any swelling that may occur in an injured lower limb on first standing upright and, it is suggested (Skinner and Thompson, 1994), aid the antigravity flow of blood and lymph to reduce oedema of the feet and ankles.

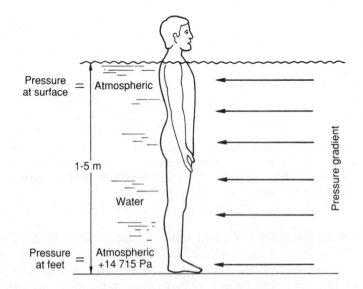

Fig. 7.1 Pressure gradient in water.

BUOYANCY

The force exerted by a fluid on an object in the fluid is equal to the weight of the fluid displaced by the object. This is Archimedes' principle. The pressure will be exerted on all immersed surfaces of the object and will depend on the sources of fluid pressure described above and, of course, be independent of the mass of the object. Thus, whether an object sinks or floats in a fluid depends on the relative densities of fluid and object.

Buoyancy is an upward force exerted on the object, which is ultimately due to the force of gravity on the surrounding fluid. An object of density less than $1000 \, kg \, m^{-3}$ will float on water because it will displace a volume of water equal to its mass. Thus a block of wood of $700 \, kg \, m^{-3}$ will float with seven-tenths of its volume immersed. An object of density greater than $1000 \, kg \, m^{-3}$ will sink in water. To remain suspended in water it is necessary to maintain an exactly equal density, which is achieved in fish by varying the amount of air in their swim bladders and, similarly, in submarines in their buoyancy tanks.

The density of the human body varies with build (notably the proportion of fat) and with the amount of air in the lungs but it is generally slightly less than that of pure water, about $980 \, kg \, m^{-3}$ is a reasonable figure. This means that the human body will float with only some 2% of it above water. Altering the buoyancy by attaching low density objects to the body – floats or a life jacket – diminishes the density of the whole object, body and float, so that a greater proportion is out of the water, making it easier to maintain the airways clear of the water. Seawater is slightly more dense than pure water so that the body will float higher.

Thus, a floating object is influenced by both the force of gravity acting downwards and the force of buoyancy acting upwards. The orientation of the floating object will depend on the interaction of these forces. Buoyancy will act through the centre of gravity of the displaced water, i.e. the centre of the volume of the object. The force of gravity will act through the centre of gravity of the object, which will not coincide with the centre of buoyancy unless the object is of uniform density. Consider the object shown in Figure 7.2, which is a piece of wood with some iron nails driven in at one end. Since the centre of gravity is much nearer the end with the nails, because of the greater density of iron, there will be a turning force exerted, as shown in Figure 7.2, so that the wood floats with one end projecting from the water and the other submerged. Designs to keep the centre of gravity of boats below the centre of buoyancy are essential to prevent capsize. When the trunk is fixed, the limbs can behave as levers with gravitational forces modified by the effect of buoyancy in the hydrotherapy pool. The idea is illustrated in Figure 7.3, in which the buoyancy of the distal part of the limb has been increased by the attachment of a float. This can be used as an assistance to raising the limb or to give resistance to depressing it. The magnitude of the turning force exerted will depend on the distance from the axis of the float, as described

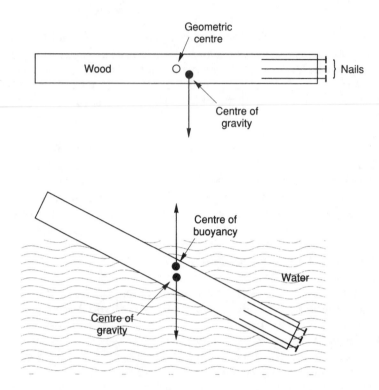

Fig. 7.2 Object of non-uniform density.

in Chapter 5. Placing the float further from the joint will increase the torque. Similarly, the torque will vary as the limb angle changes, it being greatest when the limb is at the horizontal (see Fig. 7.3).

A person standing upright, partly immersed in water, will have some of their weight supported by water, with buoyancy counteracting the normal gravitational pull. Weightbearing through the legs and feet is, therefore, reduced. This is a useful therapeutic effect, since it allows upright standing with reduced compression force through injured joints and other tissues. This has been quantified and it has been found that standing in water to the level of the anterior superior iliac spines (57% of the body immersed) leads to a reduction in weightbearing to about 50% and, with water at the level of the xiphisternum (71% of the body immersed), to a reduction in weightbearing to about 30% (Harrison and Bulstrode, 1987; Harrison *et al.*, 1992). Of course, during standing, the weight would be divided (not necessarily equally) between the two lower limbs and hence allow about half the force on one lower limb. During walking in water, these forces would be much greater due both to the push off and to the fact that at some point in the walking cycle all the weight passes through one lower limb (see Harrison *et al.*, 1992).

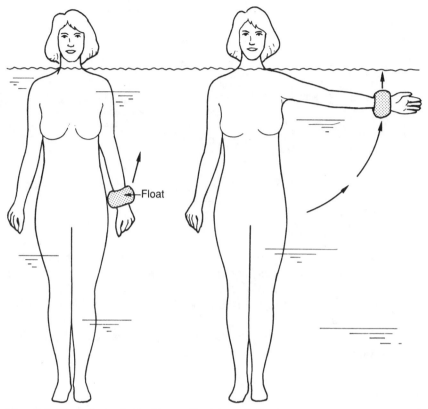

Fig. 7.3 The effect of attaching a float to a limb.

SURFACE TENSION

One further force acting in liquids is that of surface tension. Molecules exert both attraction and repulsion forces on one another, as described in Figure 2.5. In liquids, the balance of forces is such as to allow motion but not wide separation of molecules as occurs in gases. The cohesive forces of a homogeneous liquid keep the molecules in the interior of the liquid approximately the same average distance apart. Where the liquid meets a different substance – that is at a surface – the balance of forces is different. Thus, at the air/water interface the cohesive forces on water molecules are much greater than adhesive forces between water and air molecules. Consequently, water molecules at the surface are held downwards more tightly than they are pulled upwards. This results in an elastic 'skin' on the water surface formed of molecules under tension and trying to reduce the area of the surface (see Fig. 7.4). This is, of course, opposed by the pressure within the liquid and accounts for well recognized phenomena such as the near spherical shape of small water droplets and the formation of bubbles in which the inside pressure is that of a gas. At the interface between water and a more dense material such as glass, the adhesive forces between water and glass molecules are greater,

Basic Biomechanics Explained

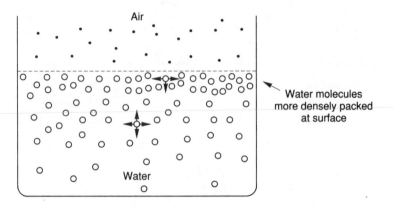

Fig. 7.4 Surface tension.

so that the water adheres to the glass. This accounts for the water droplets remaining adherent to a glass container after wetting it. It also accounts for the important mechanism of capillary action in which liquid is drawn along a narrow tube due to the strong adhesive effects of the wall of the tube on the liquid.

So far only the forces acting in fluids at rest have been considered. Fluid dynamics are much more complex.

VISCOSITY

Viscosity has already been considered in Chapter 6 and reference should be made to p. 111 and Table 6.3. Viscous force is large when the force needed to move molecules of a fluid over one another is also large. It is an intrinsic property of the fluid itself and is temperature dependent; in liquids, raising the temperature decreases viscosity.

LIQUID FLOW

The way in which liquids move is crucially dependent on their viscosity and the velocity of the flow. At low velocities the flow occurs in the manner described in Chapter 6 for lubricants, in which layers of the fluid move over one another (Fig. 6.3); hence, it is called laminar flow. At a critical velocity, dependent on the viscosity, the character of the flow changes so that it tends to move in small circles and eddies rather than in the regular layered form. This irregular flow is called turbulence. The effect is illustrated by smoke rising from the end of a cigarette at first in a column but, as it speeds up, the flow becomes turbulent. Laminar flow in pipes occurs in the way illustrated in Figure 7.5, with the outer circumferential layer of liquid in contact with the wall of the pipe hardly moving at all, while successive inner concentric layers move with progressively greater velocities. Blood flows in this way in the vessels.

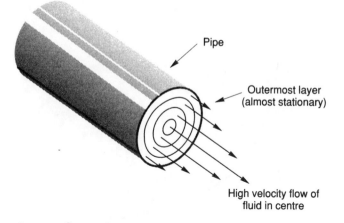

Fig. 7.5 Laminar flow in pipes.

The flow of fluid in a pipe will depend directly on the difference in pressure between the two ends and inversely on the resistance to the flow. (In the same way as the electric current in a conductor depends directly on the electromotive force and inversely on the resistance – Ohm's law – see *Physical Principles Explained*.) The flow rate in the blood vessels is, therefore, dependent on the force of the heart beat and the resistance provided by the vessels, which is known as the peripheral resistance. This resistance is due both to the viscosity of the fluid – greater viscosity will cause greater resistance – and to the ratio of the volume of fluid to the area of pipe wall with which it is in contact. Clearly, longer pipes will offer greater resistance but pipes with large cross-sections will offer lower resistance. In fact, the cross-sectional area of the pipe is by far the most important variable in that the rate of flow for a given pressure is proportional to the fourth power of the radius of the pipe. This is known as Poiseuille's law. This means that, if a blood vessel of radius 2 mm is constricted to a radius of 1 mm, the blood flow would be reduced to one sixteenth of its original value. This shows how small changes in arteriole diameter can have a dramatic effect on local blood flow. (Of course, in the body it is not as simple as suggested above; many other factors vary, notably the blood pressure.) Poiseuille's law is true for laminar flow, which occurs in blood vessels but in many other situations much turbulence occurs leading to higher resistance.

What applies to liquid moving against walls of pipes also applies to solid objects moving through liquids, like fish, humans and boats moving through water. For streamlined objects, such as fish, moving at low velocities, the flow of water over most of the surface is laminar. Irregular shapes, especially non-smooth surfaces, produce turbulence, which greatly increases the resistance to motion. The increased resistance for an object of any given shape moving in any particular liquid is approximately proportional to the square of its velocity. The nature of turbulent flow is extremely complex, involving rotational movements and other irregular

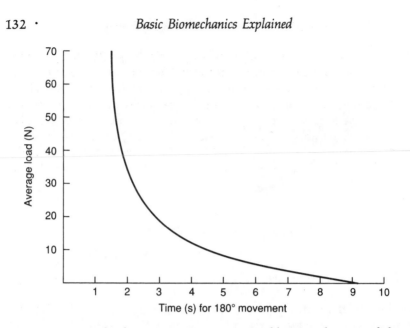

Fig. 7.6 Average load in newtons on an 18 cm table-tennis bat moved through 180° at the end of an 0.8 m limb at different velocities in water (modified from Hillman *et al.*, 1987).

motion of fluid molecules. It is considered that some of the incredible efficiency of swimming fishes arises due to their skilful reuse of energy from the turbulence they generate.

This resistance to movement through water, hydrostatic drag, is the principal way of offering resistance to exercise in the hydrotherapy pool. Since resistance increases sharply with velocity, moving slightly more quickly leads to greater resistance. The turbulence can be increased by fixing some object with a large surface area to the moving limb; a table tennis bat held in the hand is often used for the upper limb. Holding the bat with the flat face pressing against the water as the limb is swung through an arc provides very considerable resistance. This has been usefully quantified and a graph showing the average load at different speeds of moving the upper limb through 180° is shown in Figure 7.6, which is modified from Hillman *et al.* (1987). These researchers provide a clinically applicable means of quantifying the loads applied in hydrotherapy exercises. It should be understood that Figure 7.6 illustrates average loads at average speeds for a particular size of bat. Peak load can be very much greater. Hillman *et al.* found the peak load in their experiments to be approximately 1.7 times the average load.

SWIMMING

Human swimming is a very inefficient method of travel in that it uses a great deal of metabolic energy for a low-speed progress of about

$1-2\,\mathrm{m\,s^{-1}}$. This is due to the large hydrodynamic drag of the body and the relatively small surface area of the hands and feet that are used to push on the water. Increasing the area by using flippers improves efficiency. Fishes with large tail flukes are able to push large masses of water, compared with their own mass, at low velocity thus achieving much higher efficiencies. The fastest swimming stroke, the front crawl, has a world record of about 48 seconds for 100 m (just over $2\,\mathrm{m\,s^{-1}}$) and about $2.29\,\mathrm{m\,s^{-1}}$ for 50 m (Alexander, 1992), which illustrates the powerful effect of hydrostatic drag.

THE THERAPEUTIC VALUE OF WATER

The use of warm water to treat bodily ailments has a long and interesting history. The principal beneficial effects of immersion are considered to be:

1. The relief of pain induced both by the warmth of the water (38°C) and support due to buoyancy and pressure. These may be associated with relaxation.
2. The resistance to motion imposed by the water, which can be finely controlled by varying the rate of movement and utilized for muscle re-education. It also limits rapid uncontrolled movement, which helps those with some neurological deficit as well as those with joint pain.
3. The weight-relief afforded by buoyancy is useful in the re-education of lower limb injuries.
4. The freedom allowed in water for some patients whose movements on dry land are constrained. Swimming has been found to be particularly beneficial physically, as well as mentally rewarding, for many handicapped patients (Martin, 1981).

Many other effects from bathing in warm water, aside from those pertaining to exercise, have been considered therapeutically valuable, in particular the circulatory adjustments noted above.

While there is much agreement concerning the subjective benefits of exercise in water, there are few studies quantifying the improvement or comparing it with a similar, cheaper land-based exercise regimen. One such study, however, investigating treatment outcome following anterior cruciate ligament reconstruction, concluded that treatment in the hydrotherapy pool was more effective in reducing effusion and facilitating recovery of function than dry land treatment. Other outcomes, such as joint range of movement and quadriceps muscle strength, were similar, although some muscle strengthening appeared to be better promoted by land-based exercises (Tovin *et al.*, 1994). It should be noted that many normal activities, such as walking, do not exercise the same muscle groups when performed in water. This is one limitation of this therapy.

For a detailed description of the uses and techniques of hydrotherapy, reference should be made to Skinner and Thompson (1983), Reid Campion (1990), Davis and Harrison (1988), and Golland (1981).

8. *Pressure: some therapeutic applications*

Pressure is defined as force per unit area. It has already been considered in Chapter 7 in connection with fluids, in which it was noted that pressure acts in all directions and is ultimately due to both the weight of the fluid and any force acting on its surface. Pressures on solids are considered at the junctions of solid surfaces, due, for example, to the action and reaction forces considered in Chapter 2.

When a solid object at rest on a surface is considered, as someone standing with both feet on the floor, it is easy to see that the pressure between the shoe and the floor is the weight of the person divided by the area of their shoes in contact with the floor. If that area is $100\,cm^2$ for each shoe and the person weighs 60 kg, then a mass of 0.3 kg would be applied to each square centimetre. Multiplying the mass by the acceleration due to gravity of $9.8\,m\,s^{-2}$ will give the force in newtons (N), so the pressure would be $2.94\,N\,cm^{-2}$ ($0.3 \times 9.8 = 2.94$, or $29\,400\,N\,m^{-2}$). Standing on one foot doubles the pressure. Making the area of contact with the ground smaller will increase the local pressure – as occurs with football boot studs or with crampons – as noted in Chapter 6. Similarly, increasing the area of contact, as occurs with skis or snow shoes, would diminish the pressure. When standing on bare feet, the foot shape conforms to the pressure somewhat, so that the area in contact with the floor increases with all the weight on one foot and decreases when the weight is divided between the two feet again.

MEASUREMENT OF PRESSURE

Due to the different ways in which pressure has been measured historically, there are several units of pressure. The SI unit, noted in Chapter 7, is the pascal (Pa). This is quite a small unit: $1\,Pa = 1\,N\,m^{-2}$. The kilopascal (kPa) is commonly found in medical science, $1\,kPa = 1000\,Pa$. In meteorology particularly, the bar is used as a unit of pressure, $1\,bar = 100\,000\,Pa$. One thousandth of a bar is a millibar (mb), which is also commonly employed; thus, $1\,mb = 100\,Pa$.

Traditional units for measuring pressure have developed from measuring the height of a column of mercury that the pressure will support. Systolic and diastolic blood pressures, measured by means of a sphygmomanometer, are given in millimetres of mercury (mm Hg). Due to its familiarity, this method of measuring pressure is most often given when describing pressure devices dealing with tissue fluid pressure. It will be used in the following pages. This is done in the interests of clarity, conforming to the well known, but the relationships in Table 8.1 should be noted.

Atmospheric pressure is properly measured in millibars but many barometers give the pressure in mm Hg; thus, 1013 mb = 760 mm Hg.

Table 8.1 Units of pressure

Kilopascal	Pascal	Bar	mm Hg
1	1000	0.01	7.5
0.001	1	0.00001	0.0075
100	100 000	1	750
0.133	133.3	0.00133	1

PRESSURE CHANGES ON THE BODY TISSUES

The hydrostatic pressure of fluids in the tissues is necessarily influenced by the pressure outside the body, normally the atmospheric pressure, so that the gauge pressure is actually measured (see Chapter 7). It is the balance between the blood and extracellular tissue (interstitial fluid) pressures that allows the exchange of fluid between these two compartments and with intracellular fluid. Even quite small changes in atmospheric pressure – especially if they occur abruptly – can affect the tissue fluid exchange. Thus, the lowered pressures that occur during air travel coupled with lack of movement and the dependent position can lead to swelling of the feet. It is considered that the increased pain in many chronic conditions associated with changes in the weather may be due to the relatively rapid changes in barometric pressure associated with weather fronts.

THE USE OF PRESSURE FOR THERAPY

Manual massage is the best known and most ancient use of varying pressure for therapeutic purposes. The techniques and effects are described in other texts. The effect of water pressure on the body was noted in Chapter 7. Mechanical pressure is also applied to the skin surface, both continuously and intermittently, for therapeutic purposes. Continuous or semicontinuous pressure is applied to the tissue by bandages or pressure garments. Negative pressure (suction) and positive pressure (compression) are both applied intermittently with cycles of a few minutes for therapy.

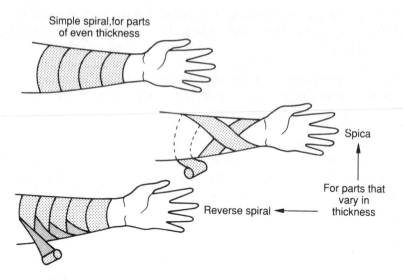

Simple spiral,for parts
of even thickness

Spica

For parts that
vary in
thickness

Reverse spiral ◄———

Fig. 8.1 Forms of bandaging.

When pressure is applied at higher frequencies – a few hertz to around
100 Hz – it is commonly called vibration when applied locally and
shaking if applied to larger areas.

Continuous pressure

Continuous pressure is widely used therapeutically for the control of
oedema by means of bandages wrapped around the part. It is important to
generate an even force over the whole surface of the tissues and not allow
a greater pressure to be applied to one area causing a constriction. This
problem is obviated in various ways. The use of elastic material for the
bandage, such as crepe, allows the bandage to conform to the shape of the
part while maintaining uniform pressure. The pressure is provided by the
recoil of the elastic, which is slightly stretched while being applied. The
use of padding beneath the bandage or between layers of the bandage
spreads the tension force more evenly. The Robert Jones compression
bandage is an example in which thick layers of cotton wool separate two
or three layers of bandage. Applying the bandage spirally avoids
circumferential constrictions and allows the bandage to conform to the
shape of the limb, providing it is of even circumference. The reason for
using spicas, or better still reverse spirals, is that the two edges of the
bandage travel the same distance over parts that vary in circumference
(see Fig. 8.1).

Similar compression effects can be achieved very conveniently by using
a tubular elastic bandage. Versions of this bandage and elastic stockings or
sleeves, which are shaped to fit the limb, are likely to be rather more

effective when they are made to measure for the patient because they conform to the exact shape and thus produce uniform pressure throughout the limb.

Pressure applied by bandages serves to control tissue oedema and thus needs to balance the interstitial pressure. Bandages can be applied to give pressures of 25–50 mm Hg (Thomas *et al.*, 1981). The pressure generated depends on the method of application, the number of layers of bandage, the radius of curvature – a smaller limb diameter leads to higher pressure – and the elasticity of the bandage. The elasticity of bandages is due to the twisting of threads in the weave, except for special bandages, blue line webbing for instance, which have some rubber or elastic material incorporated into the fabric. These latter are especially suitable for providing compression and are often used in the treatment of varicose veins and obstructive oedema. The various categories of bandages are given in Table 8.2.

Table 8.2 Categories of bandages

Type of bandage	Examples	Uses	Tension/pressure
Crepe	Crepe bandage	Mild compression Restricts movement Secures dressings	
Cotton crepe	Elastocrepe Creban cotton crepe Crevic	As above	Low tension/ light pressure
Cotton stretch	Creban cotton stretch Grip Sanicrepe	Secures dressings mainly	
Elastic	Blue line webbing Red line webbing Elset	Compression, for control of oedema	High tension/ firm pressure

It has been found (Thomas *et al.*, 1981) that when the crepe, cotton crepe and cotton stretch bandages are applied by experienced staff, initial pressures on a limb are between 51 and 67 mm Hg, but this would be expected to fall gradually (on average by about 40% in 20 minutes) to maintain a constant pressure. In spite of wide variations from one bandage to another, the staff were able to compensate to produce a remarkably consistent set of pressures. In fact, there seems to be little difference between these groups of bandages. However, the elastic bandages can provide higher initial pressures, at about 80 mm Hg, which is well maintained (falling 17% in 20 minutes).

Knitted tubular bandages are widely used to provide compression.

These are convenient and effective, providing the appropriate size and number of layers to give adequate pressure are used. It is essential that the proximal ends of the limb tubes are not allowed to roll over and cause constriction.

It would seem that the effectiveness of a bandage in providing an appropriate degree of compression is more dependent on the skill of the person applying the bandage than on its physical characteristics.

Direct compression is used in the treatment and prevention of hypertrophic scarring. The scar is held in a stretched position and compressed by a moulded plastic splint, held in place by firm elastic bandaging (George, 1975), or special elastic garments can be provided. To be effective, pressure must be maintained almost continuously over several months. It is considered that the prevention of oedema in, and the reduced vascularity of, the scar are the key factors in preventing hypertrophy.

Negative pressure devices

Local suction has been used therapeutically for many centuries; it was known as cupping. It was probably popular because it combined the appealing idea of 'drawing out poisons' with painless skin stimulation while leaving visible dramatic evidence of the effect in the form of a ring of erythema that persisted after removal of the cup. It was often performed by pressing warmed copper or glass cups on to the skin so that a mild suction was produced as the air cooled and contracted.

The modern version of this therapy is found in the use of suction to fix the electrodes for applying interferential therapy. Mild suction is applied through tubes to a flexible rubber cup, which contains both the electrode and a wet sponge pad. The suction must be sufficient to maintain good contact between the sponge and the skin. On the other hand, suction must not be so strong as to cause skin damage, since interferential treatments are often applied for 20 minutes or more. The negative suction pressures used are in the region of −150 to −500 mm Hg (−0.2 to −0.7 bar). Most units vary the suction automatically in cycles of a few seconds to further diminish any risk of bruising and provide gentle massaging to the skin. As well as holding the electrodes in place, this mild suction causes vasodilation, which may lower the electrical resistance of the skin. The stimulation of sensory nerves affecting the pain gate mechanism and the increased cutaneous blood flow may be beneficial to the condition being treated (see *Electrotherapy Explained*, 2nd edition).

Positive pressure devices

Probably the earliest, and certainly the simplest, positive pressure device was the roller. This essentially consists of a smooth or corrugated roller, or

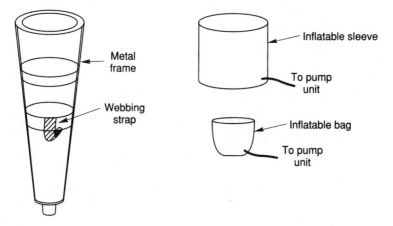

Fig. 8.2 Pneumatic postamputation mobility (PPAM) aid.

sometimes a set of wheels or spheres, mounted on an axle, which is pushed over the skin with an appropriate degree of pressure exerted through a handle. Many versions of 'roller massagers', made from different materials have been popular over the years. Recently, wooden ones have reappeared. They are rolled over the skin with a firm pressure, either to and fro or with repeated strokes in the same direction, with sufficient pressure to depress the tissues beneath the roller. Apart from sensory stimulation and the massaging effects of local pressure, there seems to be no specific therapeutic effect.

The best known positive pressure devices involve controlled air pressure applied to the limb by some form of large cuff to provide compression around the limb or as varied pressure pads and mattresses.

The pneumatic postamputation mobility (PPAM) aid

This is an early partial weightbearing aid for use after above and below knee amputations. It consists of a frame and two inflatable air bags, which surround the stump (see Fig. 8.2). It can be used in the physiotherapy department within a few days postoperatively, providing the wound is healing well. The use of the PPAM aid varies from standing briefly in parallel bars to approximately two hours of walking, standing and resting. During rest periods, the large bag is deflated and the stump and PPAM aid elevated. Younger and more able patients can progress to partial weightbearing with crutches on level ground. Two PPAM aids should not be used for bilateral amputations.

Intermittent pneumatic compression

An arm or a leg is encased in an air bag, which can be inflated by a pump to a predetermined pressure and then released. The timing of each phase

Basic Biomechanics Explained

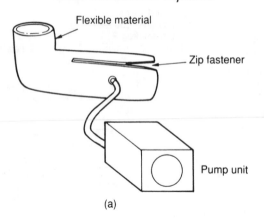

(a)

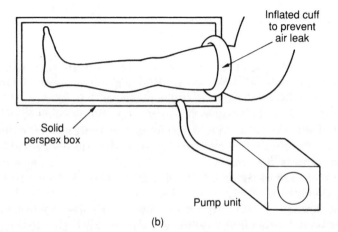

(b)

Fig. 8.3 Positive pressure devices: (a) intermittent positive pressure; (b) vacuum compression therapy.

of the pressure–release cycle is controlled by the machine. The pressure garments are often made of a tough pliable airtight material such as polyurethane reinforced nylon.

In the most commonly employed type, the garment is a single compartment boot or sleeve, which can be opened along the front by a zip fastener for easy insertion of the limb. The fingers or toes are usually left exposed (see Fig. 8.3a). In the simplest versions, a fixed cycle lasting a few minutes is used during which the garment alternately inflates to a chosen pressure and then deflates to zero. More sophisticated machines provide the means of altering both inflation and deflation pressures as well as wide variations in the cycle times. For a comparison of the performance of some of these machines see Rithalia *et al.* (1987) and Sayegh *et al.* (1987). Some machines have a means of controlling the pressure electronically and timing the cycles so that once set (programmed) the treatment can be repeated subsequently without need of further adjustment.

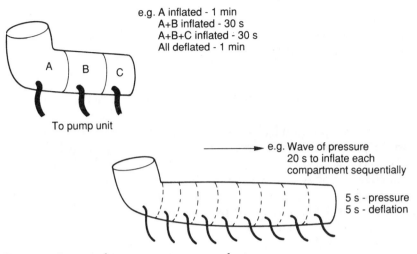

Fig. 8.4 Sequential intermittent pressure devices.

A different device consists of a rigid cylinder – often made of perspex – into which the limb is fitted, being sealed by a proximally placed cuff. Since the enclosing cylinder is rigid, both positive and negative pressure can be applied by air pumped into or out of the container in a cyclical manner. This has been called 'vacuum compression therapy' (see Fig. 8.3b).

The application of air pressure to the tissues inside a clear plastic bag may be called pneumotherapy. Both single bags, in which the air is blown directly between the plastic bag and the skin – sometimes called pulsed environmental therapy – and double bags are used (Salter, 1987).

A somewhat more complex system, which simulates manual massage to some extent, uses a pressure garment divided into a number of compartments. These are inflated sequentially so that pressure is applied first at the end of the limb and then more proximally. The distal bags remain inflated until all segments are fully inflated, at which point they all deflate simultaneously (see Fig. 8.4). These systems have been called sequential intermittent pneumatic compression devices (see Sayegh *et al.,* 1987).

PHYSIOLOGICAL EFFECTS AND THERAPEUTIC USES

As the different devices described above have very similar effects, they will be considered together. The basic effect of intermittent pneumatic compression is to squeeze blood and lymph proximally in their soft-walled vessels, in the same manner as the normal physiological muscle pump works, back flow being prevented by the valves. If the limb is oedematous, the external force raises the pressure so that there is greater transfer from tissue fluid to blood (Sayegh *et al.,* 1987). As a result of these effects, it would be expected that the formation of thrombi in the veins would be prevented to some degree and oedema diminished. Both of these effects have been demonstrated.

Prevention of deep vein thrombosis (DVT)

Intermittent compression has been recommended and applied to the leg in order to prevent the occurrence of DVT for many years (Clark *et al.*, 1974). Hills *et al.* (1972) found it to be successful in a double-blind trial, in which compression was applied to the calf during surgery and for the first two postoperative days. Quite a low inflation pressure of 40 mm Hg applied for 15 s with a 45 s or 60 s deflation period has been recommended as the optimal for the prevention of DVT by continuous application (Sayegh *et al.*, 1987).

This success in the prevention of DVT is considered to be due to three mechanisms (Sayegh *et al.*, 1987). First, stasis in the valve pockets is prevented due to the increased peak blood flow in the veins. Each time the limb is squeezed, a larger and more rapid flow occurs. Secondly, if fast cycles are used, the mean blood flow increases, and, thirdly, this treatment increases fibrinolysis, possibly by encouraging the formation or distribution of a fibinolytic activator substance produced in the vein walls. This may account for the finding that intermittent compression of the arm reduces the incidence of DVT in the legs (Knight and Dawson, 1976).

Reduction of oedema

Limb swelling is very often due to either venous or lymphatic obstruction or the late consequence of venous thrombosis, or occurs after the lymph nodes have been destroyed by radiation or surgery in the treatment of breast cancer. There is good evidence showing that intermittent compression helps to reduce limb swelling in these patients (Gray, 1987; Gillham, 1994). Clearly, both increasing the interstitial fluid pressure to encourage fluid into the capillaries, and increasing the venous and lymphatic flow, are likely to help to reduce the oedema. It has been suggested (Sayegh *et al.*, 1987) on theoretical grounds that pressure should be kept below capillary pressure (about 10 mm Hg), with the patient in supine lying and at about 40 mm Hg in half lying, so that the capillaries are not occluded. Most therapists, however, use rather higher pressures.

As a consequence of greater venous blood flow and oedema reduction, there are other therapeutic benefits. These include accelerated wound healing, less fluid collection in wounds and reduced haematoma formation. Intermittent compression has been used after limb surgery and in the treatment of venous leg ulcers. Pneumotherapy is valuable in the treatment of hand oedema; it is safe and hand movements can be practised since the part can be seen through the plastic container.

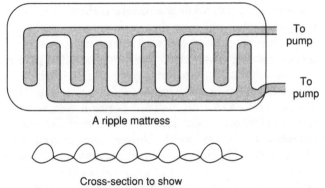

A ripple mattress

Cross-section to show
alternate cells inflated
and deflated

Fig. 8.5 Alternating pressure surfaces.

Alternating pressure surfaces for the prevention and treatment of pressure sores

These are well known and widely used in the form of 'ripple mattresses' and 'ripple pressure pads'. Pressure sores develop in areas where long periods of compression of the patient's tissues occur, usually between a bony point and the surface on which the individual is lying or sitting. This will only happen if the tissues are in a poor nutritional state, as in uncontrolled diabetes, or, importantly, when there is sensory loss. Other risk factors are immobility, deformity, drug abuse, obesity and urine-soaked skin. If the patient cannot alter the position of the body relative to the surface on which they are sitting or lying, the surface is made to alter under them. This is effected by means of a series of air cells or tubes forming the mattress or pad. Alternate cells are inflated with air for two minutes or so and then allowed to deflate while the intervening cells are inflated (see Fig. 8.5). There are numerous versions of this idea, forming wheelchair pads and mattresses, which are invaluable for those with permanent sensory loss, such as paraplegics.

Assessment and diagnostic devices

The measurement of pressure can be extremely valuable in assessment and monitoring the effects of treatment. The following are examples.

1. Muscle strength can be assessed by means of a myometer, as described in Chapter 5, which measures the pressure generated between the patient's limb and the tester's hand as the patient attempts movement.
2. The pressure in various sites between the patient and the seat of a chair can be measured. This is valuable to assess the risk of pressure

sores arising on the skin of a patient with sensory loss who is using a wheelchair.
3. A perineometer also works by measuring pressure. This is used in female patients to measure the strength of the pelvic floor muscles for assessment and encouragement during their re-education. The sensor is placed in the vagina.
4. Pressure of the foot on the floor can be measured by a flat device in the shoe, known as a limb load monitor. This is useful for the assessment of load on the lower limb in gait re-education and assessment. The force plate was described in Chapter 3.

In some of these instruments, air is compressed by the force being tested and the air pressure is directly measured by a mechanical pressure gauge. In others, the electrical output from a piezo-electrical crystal device – a transducer – is displayed on a meter. Sometimes air pressure is used to transmit force to the electrical sensor.

RAPID INTERMITTENT PRESSURE CHANGES

These are better understood as vibration and shaking. In some respects the effects of vibration parallel those of electrical pulses of similar frequency in that they stimulate peripheral nerves (see *Electrotherapy Explained*). At appropriate frequencies (30–20 000 Hz) vibration is recognized as sound, (see *Physical Principles Explained*) and at megahertz frequencies as ultrasound.

Vibration

Vibration refers to rapid to and fro movements. If it is being applied to large parts of the body, such as whole body segments, it is used synonymously with shaking. If it is applied locally with significant force, it is synonymous with percussion.

Devices to shake up or vibrate the whole body have a long and fascinating history. From the eighteenth century onwards, assorted mechanical devices were made, often copied from natural activities such as horse riding. A mechanical horse was made and recommended to 'shake up the liver'. Many similar machines have been produced and marketed over the years, the modern descendants being, perhaps, machines that vibrate a flexible belt or strap, which is passed around the standing subject's waist or gluteal region. Claims have been made that rapid vibration will 'break down' fat in these regions. Not surprisingly, there is no evidence, other than anecdotal, for this effect. Whole body 'shakers' tend to work at 1–2 Hz, whereas the vibrating belts (which have often been called 'oscillators') often work at around 5 Hz.

Modern hand-held mechanical vibrators are used to produce local vibration or to percuss the part. They work at frequencies of anything between 20 and 300 Hz, but mostly at around 50 Hz or 100 Hz. They can be considered in two groups. First are the mains operated types, with a rubber or hard plastic applicator of about 5 cm diameter driven by an electric motor via a mechanical linkage, which makes the applicator vibrate. Secondly, there are small battery operated devices with smaller applicators, which work with much lower force but at similar frequencies to the mains type. These will, however, stimulate sensory nerves when applied to the skin.

Many devices for 'vibratory massage' to particular areas have been made, for example, vibrating pillows for the back and neck. These are mostly mains operated and sold to the public.

Measurement of vibration

The parameters of vibration or percussion treatments are the frequency, as noted already, the amplitude of motion of the applicator, and the acceleration (rate of change of velocity) of the applicator. In general, the amplitude (displacement of the applicator as it vibrates) is greater with the large machines. For most hand-held vibrators, it is of the order of a few millimetres. The acceleration of these vibrators is likely to be below $1 \, \text{m} \, \text{s}^{-2}$, although there is little published information.

9. Human movement: description and analysis including gait

INTRODUCTION

Motion is often described as translatory, in order to depict a non-reciprocating movement of matter or a body from one place to another. This may involve linear motion, when all parts of the body or object move the same distance in the same direction and in the same time. It may also involve angular or rotary motion in which the body moves about a fixed point so that all parts of the body move through the same angular displacement. The trajectory of a projectile may be described as curvilinear motion. The concept of the motion of a body is distinguished from that of the body being at rest. This is often ambiguous because the body can be moving as part of one system, while at rest with respect to another. Thus, the velocity of the forward swing of the arm during walking might be described with respect to the trunk, but would be greater if described with respect to the ground because of the forward motion of the walker. If the walk were being taken in the aisle of an aircraft travelling at, say, 600 mph, then the velocity with respect to the surface of the earth is again very different. An observer in space would give a different answer again because of the motion of the earth. Thus motion is described in a particular frame of reference. It may be noted that if the frame of reference is moving at a constant velocity (uniform motion) – i.e. there are no changes in speed or direction – it exerts no forces on the object. It is only when the aircraft is climbing or accelerating that the seated passenger is aware of motion (see Chapter 1: Newton's first law).

Velocity is a vector quantity, like force or displacement, which have both their magnitude and direction specified. Scalar quantities, such as mass, time, temperature and speed, have only magnitude and can be added or subtracted arithmetically. Vectors, on the other hand, since they involve direction, must be handled in a special way. Consider the velocity of a parachutist descending at $7 \, \text{m s}^{-1}$ (compare Fig. 6.4b) but affected by a wind blowing horizontally at a velocity of $4 \, \text{m s}^{-1}$ as indicated in Figure 9.1. It is easy to see that, since the force of gravity is acting vertically while the force of the wind is acting horizontally, the resulting direction will be the hypotenuse of a right angle triangle. If the other sides are drawn in proportion to the magnitude of the vectors (speeds), as in Figure 9.1, the length of the hypotenuse is also in proportion.

What is usually described is the average or mean velocity, since the actual velocity for each time unit – each minute or each second – might

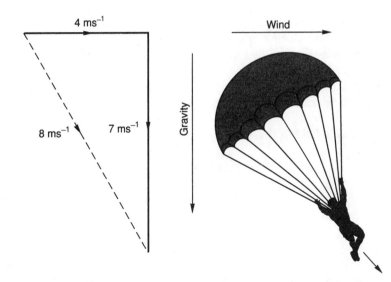

Fig. 9.1 Parachutist falling due to gravity and affected by the force of the wind: falling vertically at $7\,\text{m s}^{-1}$ and moving sideways with a velocity of $4\,\text{m s}^{-1}$; vectors can be added graphically in the triangle drawn to scale. (Note: $4^2 + 7^2$ (65) $= 8^2$ (64)).

differ. Velocity is simply the displacement per unit time (or speed in a given direction), so the velocity at any instant can vary.

Displacement, which is also a vector quantity, describes the separation of two points in terms of both the distance travelled and the direction. During walking, the centre of gravity of the human body may move, say, 20 metres in a northerly direction – the displacement – but to do so it follows a slightly sinuously curved path as the body moves up and down at each step, as will be described. If this walk takes 30 s then the average velocity would be $1.5\,\text{m s}^{-1}$, but the average speed of the centre of gravity would be a little greater because it travels a slightly greater distance.

ACCELERATION

Whenever the velocity of a body changes, either in magnitude or direction, the change is an acceleration. This may be an increase or a decrease, or positive or negative acceleration. Negative acceleration is also described as deceleration or retardation. Since it is the change in velocity per unit time, it will be measured in units of distance per unit time per unit time i.e. metres per second per second (m s^{-2}). It will also be a vector quantity.

For uniform acceleration, the relationships between its velocity and displacement are given by four equations. The customary symbols used are:

u for the initial velocity in $m\,s^{-1}$
v for the final velocity also in $m\,s^{-1}$
t for the time in s
a for the acceleration in $m\,s^{-2}$
s for distance covered in m

The equations linking these are

$$v = u + at \tag{1}$$

$$s = ut + \tfrac{1}{2}\,at^2 \tag{2}$$

$$s = \tfrac{1}{2}(ut + vt) \tag{3}$$

$$v^2 = u^2 + 2as \tag{4}$$

For a body starting from rest, i.e. with no initial velocity, u would be zero. Consider the sky diver of Chapter 6 (Fig. 6.4a). Initially the drag due to air resistance would be so small that it can be ignored, so that from Equation (1) it can be seen that he would be falling with a velocity of $9.8\,m\,s^{-1}$ after the first second:

$$v = 0 + 9.81\,m\,s^{-2} \times 1$$

and a velocity of $19.62\,m\,s^{-1}$ after 2 seconds.

Similarly, Equation (2) shows:

$$s = 0 + \tfrac{1}{2} \times 9.81 \times 1$$

(s = 4.9 m which is the distance fallen after 1 second) and

$$s = 0 + \tfrac{1}{2} \times 9.81 \times 4$$

(s = 19.62 m which is the distance fallen after 2 seconds).

For a falling body, e.g. the sky-diver, if air friction is ignored, the graphs of acceleration, velocity and displacement against time are as shown in Figure 9.2.

Descriptions of body movement involve considerations of forces, which are given by the product of mass and acceleration, as described in Chapter 1. Consider a standing jump in which both knees are bent and then rapidly straightened, so that the subject leaps into the air raising their centre of gravity a distance of, say 30 cm. What is the velocity at take off? Knowing the distance (s) was 0.3 m and the final velocity (v) was zero, the acceleration due to gravity (a) acting against the movement is $9.81\,m\,s^{-2}$, so Equation (4) can be used:

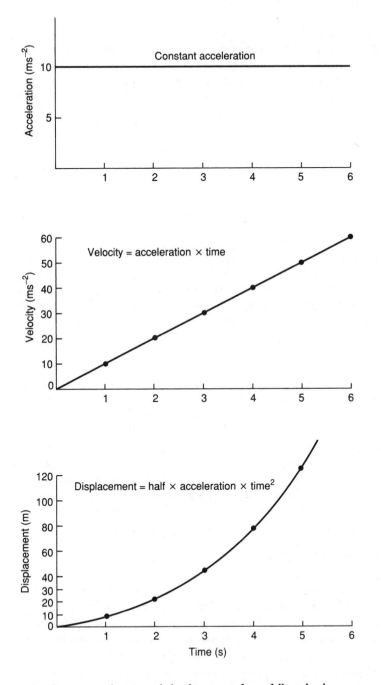

Fig. 9.2 Acceleration, velocity and displacement for a falling body.

$$v^2 = u^2 + 2as$$
$$0 = u^2 + 2(-9.81 \times 0.3)$$
$$0 = u^2 - 5.886$$
$$u = 2.4261 \text{ m s}^{-1}$$

This is about 8.734 km per h or just under 5.5 mph. In order to achieve this velocity, what acceleration from rest is needed and over what period of time would it be applied?

To take off from a crouching position, the centre of gravity moves through, say, half a metre. Applying the same equation with the initial velocity (u) now zero, the final velocity (v) found to be 2.4261 m s^{-1} and a distance of 0.5 m:

$$v^2 = u^2 + 2as$$
$$(2.4261)^2 = 0 + 2a \times 0.5$$
$$5.886 = a$$

Using Equation (1):

$$v = u + at$$
$$2.4261 = 0 + 5.886 \times t$$
$$0.4122 = t$$

To achieve this acceleration during approximately 0.4 s, the lower limb must be extended with appropriate force. This can be found for any given mass from the fact that F = ma (see Chapter 1). Thus, a 50 kg woman making this jump would need to exert a force of:

$$50 \times 5.886 = 294.3 \text{ N}$$

This force of about 300 N would, of course, be divided between the two lower limbs and generated principally by the extensor muscles of the hip and knee joints, together with the ankle plantarflexors. Force plate records for athletes jumping as high as possible showed the maximum force possible is about twice the body weight (Alexander, 1992), i.e. about 981 N for the 50 kg woman. Various simplifying assumptions have been made in this example. A significant omission is the contribution of the arms, which are swung rapidly upwards during such a jump. Jumping mechanisms are considered again later in this chapter.

ROTARY MOTION

Motion around an axis, or rotary motion, involves not only a change of position but also continuously changing direction. Thus, in swinging the extended upper limb at the axis of the shoulder joint, the hand travels through an arc of a certain length and the elbow through the same arc but a shorter linear distance. The identical angular changes, continually changing direction, can be described in degrees (as in Chapter 6) or in radians. The radian is the ratio of the circumference of the arc to the

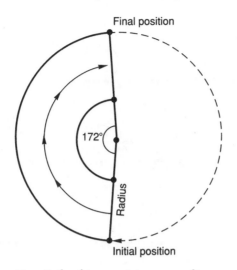

Fig. 9.3 Rotary motion: Path of two points on a radius sweeping through an angle of 172° − 3 radians − in the direction shown.

Distance around circumference between initial and final position divided by length of radius = the angle in radians (in this case, 3 radians).

Same length divided by time taken gives the linear velocity; divided by radius it gives the angular velocity in rad s^{-1}.

Linear acceleration over same length divided by the radius gives the angular velocity in rad s^{-2}.

radius. When the two are equal the ratio is one; hence, one radian is approximately equivalent to an angle of 57°; 360° is 2π radians, so that a circle is approximately 6.28 radians. This is a supplementary SI unit, which is useful for calculations relating angular and linear motions. Continuous rotation, e.g. of a wheel, can also be expressed in revolutions per unit time. Both the hand and the elbow will move through the same angle, expressed either in radians or in degrees, during the same period of time and will, therefore, have the same angular velocity. They will, of course, have different linear velocities, that of the hand being greater because it travels a greater distance in the same period of time (see Fig. 9.3). Just as the angle in radians can be found by dividing the length of the arc traversed by the radius, so the angular velocity measured in rad s^{-1} (radians per second) can be found by dividing the linear velocity by the radius (see Fig. 9.3). Similarly, the linear acceleration around the arc divided by the radius will give the angular acceleration in rad s^{-2}.

CONSERVATION OF MOMENTUM

Momentum is simply mass multiplied by velocity, as noted in Chapter 1. It can also be expressed as force multiplied by time. If one body having

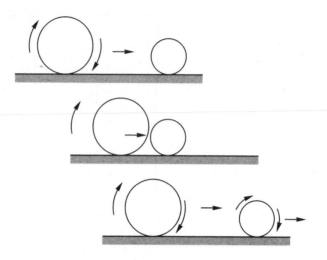

Fig. 9.4 Collision between moving objects.

momentum is driven into another body, the momentum is shared between them. This is often described for simplification in terms of moving balls of different masses striking one another, as below, but the effect is universal for the interactions of moving objects, a foot striking a ball for example, or when the objects are connected to one another as parts of the same system, as the body segments.

Consider a large, heavy ball rolled along a smooth surface to strike a stationary small, light ball (see Fig. 9.4). The force exerted by the heavy ball on the light one is exactly the same as that exerted by the light ball on the heavy one, and will act for the same length of time; the only difference will be direction. Thus, the forward momentum imparted to the light ball, in accordance with Newton's second law, is exactly equal to that lost by the heavy ball. Due to its greater mass, the large ball does not lose all forward motion so that, after the collision, both balls continue rolling in the same direction. What needs to be understood is that the momentum of the whole system – both balls – has not altered. What is lost by one ball has been gained by the other; hence the conservation of momentum. This would apply equally well to two objects connected together but able to move with respect to one another, as occurs in the limb and trunk segments of the body. Naturally, in any real system, not all the energy is conserved as mechanical energy. Some is converted to heat at each energy change or collision. Thus, allowance has to be made for this randomized energy.

The momentum of the moving body described above depends only on the mass and velocity in this linear system. In rotary motion, the same applies, but the way in which the mass is distributed relative to the axis must be additionally considered. Imagine turning a long pole held at its centre so that the two ends sweep through large horizontal or vertical arcs and compare this with the little effort needed to rotate the pole about its own longitudinal axis. In both cases, the same mass is being rotated, but in the first case much of the mass is at a considerable distance from the axis of rotation and thus must move at a higher velocity. Thus, angular momentum depends not only on velocity and mass, like linear momentum, but also on exactly where the mass is located in the rotating system. It is familiar in a heavy-rimmed flywheel, which is much harder to stop than a wheel with the same mass situated close to the hub when they are turning at the same velocity. This reluctance to change the rate of rotation is called the moment of inertia and is measured in $kg\,m^2$. Angular momentum is thus the product of the moment of inertia and angular velocity, having units of $kg\,m^2\,s^{-1}$ or $N\,m\,s$, just as the product of mass and velocity defines linear momentum in $kg\,m\,s^{-1}$.

Just as linear momentum is conserved when an object collides with another, so is angular momentum. The linear momentum of a completely isolated object cannot change velocity, but an isolated rotating body can change its own velocity. This is often dramatically seen during skilled ice dancing when the skater is seen to speed up the rotation by bringing the arms closer to the body. Due to conservation of angular momentum, when the moment of inertia is reduced by moving the mass of the arms closer to the axis of rotation, the angular velocity must increase to compensate. This, and the reverse effect of diminution in angular velocity as a consequence of moving part of the body mass further from the axis, occur in many body activities, although less obviously than in the case of the skater. The effect can be experienced with an appropriate turntable; a rotating office chair or universal balance board can be used but with appropriate care regarding the effect of rotation on the vestibular apparatus (see Chapter 3). With the subject sitting on the turntable with weights held in the outstretched hands (to increase the mass), it is set spinning and the arms and weights are suddenly brought close to the body, which is the axis of movement. It will be apparent that rotation speeds up at once. If the arms and weights are again stretched out, the speed of rotation decreases. The forces affecting these changes can be sensed in the shoulders with suitably large weights and rates of rotation.

For the human body as a whole, the moment of inertia for vertical axis rotating or twisting movements, like the spinning skater, is very much smaller than that for somersaulting about a horizontal axis through the pelvis because more mass is at a greater distance from the axis. Twists and somersaults can be made to occur during diving because the body is given angular momentum by an appropriate choice of the angle of take off; also, arm and leg movements can exchange angular momentum from one body axis to another.

It may be wondered how any person or animal can alter their position while falling without any initial angular momentum. It is well known that cats, for example, when falling out of trees will always turn in the air to land on their feet. The cat rotates its hind parts in the opposite direction to the head and forelegs about a horizontal axis during the fall. It is able to alter the moment of inertia of each part by altering the leg and head position so that a subsequent rotation brings the two parts back into line but in a new position. The cat has behaved like two separate objects; at no time does the total cat have any angular momentum.

Not only is the magnitude of angular momentum conserved in isolated systems but so is the direction. Apart from the direction of rotation – clockwise or anticlockwise, depending on the position of the observer – the direction can be defined as being along the axis of rotation. This is thoroughly familiar as the effect that keeps a spinning top or gyroscope upright. It is also part of the explanation of why it is easy to balance on a rotating bicycle wheel but very difficult when the cycle is stationary. Holding the axle of a rapidly spinning cycle wheel can demonstrate the strength of this inertial force.

DESCRIPTION AND ANALYSIS OF HUMAN MOTION

Kinetics and *Kinematics* are terms used in the analysis of human movement. While the former is sometimes used synonymously with dynamics it is often restricted to the study of mass, force and acceleration witkout concern for the position or orientation of the bodies involved. Kinematics is concerned with the study of motion, without reference to the forces involved. It is, therefore, largely descriptive. A study of biomechanical phenomena must involve both aspects because, as might be expected, there is considerable overlap. The term 'kinetics' refers to studying the role of body movements (other than speech) for communication, shoulder shrugging, winking and hand gestures, for example.

Describing human motion is a very difficult activity if complete biomechanical analysis is desired. A number of body segments are moving in three spatial dimensions with respect to one another at varying velocities and accelerations, and exerting varying forces, all of which need to be specified for a full description. It is reasonable to divide the descriptive methods into two broad groups: first, those that employ linguistic and symbolic descriptions and, secondly, those that utilize pictorial and technical means. This latter group would include not only video and cinematic recordings but graphs and other technical data derived from them.

Linguistic and notation descriptions

At the simplest level, human movement can be described to some degree by the use of normal non-specialized language; 'walking quickly' or 'making a fist' conjure up recognizable movement behaviours. To improve the description and make it applicable to less common activities will involve the use of precise anatomical terminology. This would be entirely familiar to physiotherapists. For example, the final posture of the power grip may be described by saying 'the fingers are flexed around an object, the thumb providing counter pressure through the pulp or medial border pressing against the object. The wrist is extended and ulnar deviated'. This provides only postural information and gives no information on how the position was achieved or what muscle forces are involved in maintaining it. To provide this, further extensive descriptions are needed, say, 'starting from a position with the wrist and digits fully extended and the fingers and thumb spread widely apart, the fist is rapidly clenched around the object. This activity involves concentric contraction of the finger and thumb flexor muscles as well as isometric contraction of the wrist extensors to stabilize the wrist and carpal joints'. Apart from the evident fact that this description ignores the necessary activities of other body segments, the arm and forearm, it is deficient in nominating all the muscles involved or the forces generated. The word 'rapidly' was used to give some subjective idea of the velocity of the movement.

Various written notations have been developed in an attempt to achieve a convenient method of description and communication of movement. Exercise therapists have for many years used a formalized system of abbreviations to describe the starting positions and movements involved in formal exercises. The four basic positions are standing (st.), lying (ly.), sitting (sitt.) and kneeling (kn.). Sometimes, hanging (by the arms!) was included as a starting position. From these, modifications made with altered positions of the arms and legs – called 'derived positions' – are described by adding adjectives with special meanings, such as 'yard' (yd.), denoting the arms being outstreched horizontally at the sides or 'crook' (crk.), meaning the knees are flexed. For the movement, anatomical terms, flexion, abduction etc., as well as informal words like 'bending' or 'swinging' are used, abbreviated to the first few letters. The parts of the body moved are denoted by a capital initial letter and successive letters as needed, e.g. A. = arms; Ank. = ankles. Further letters indicating direction – f. = forward, b. = backward etc. – coupled with rules controlling the order in which the abbreviations are used, allows a full description of a simple exercise. Thus 'wg.std.st.;T.bend.s.' translates as: standing with feet apart and hands on hips (wing stride standing) bending the trunk to the side (trunk bending sideways). Such a system is limited in the kind of exercise that can be described and it has to be modified by adding descriptive notes on matters like the rate and range of the movement in many practical situations. Further, the 'code' has to be thoroughly familiar to users for efficient and rapid communication of the exercise. For a full description see Gardiner (1981).

Some written notations were developed in connection with choreography, such as Benesh movement notation, which uses special symbols on a five-line musical stave. The changes of position are represented by lines drawn to indicate the direction of movement. It is claimed to be able to condense large amounts of information in such a way that these data are easily available to those skilled in the use of the system. It has been

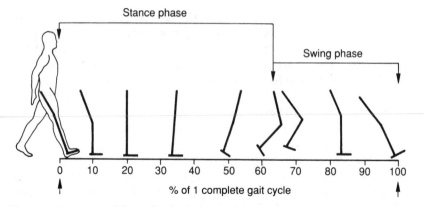

Fig. 9.5 Tracings of the right thigh, leg and foot made from a series of frames of video or film.

utilized in some clinical and research situations (McGuiness-Scott, 1982). Other notation systems have been described that are intended as universal writing systems for movement applicable to all disciplines. The use of strictly verbal descriptions of movement has been examined (Halkberg, 1976), which, while showing some consistency in that different observers tended to characterize particular movement behaviours with similar adjectives/adverbs, gave a limited number of movement categories. The reliability of all these systems seems not to have been tested. Such systems are entirely observational and can be applied directly to the movement or, more conveniently, to a video recording of the movement.

Pictorial and technical descriptions

It has already been noted that biomechanical research was given a significant boost by the invention of cinematography. Much analysis of body movement has been conducted by taking motion picture sequences, which can then be examined and analysed frame by frame. Due to the enormous amount of information in such pictures, some simplifying method is often employed. Tracings may be made of the picture in each frame to show the body segments as single straight lines, so rendering the changing angles between the segments easier to see. Such tracings are often made to illustrate normal gait; see Figure 9.5 as an example. The changed velocity of movement in different parts of the walking cycle can be seen, and, with a knowledge of the frame frequency, fairly exact estimations of these velocities can be made. A similar series of positions can be recorded by the use of reflective tape affixed to the subject moving in a darkened room while the camera shutter remains open. A light flashes at a regular frequency (stroboscopic light), recording the reflective strips all on the same film in successive positions separated by intervals corresponding to the flash frequency. This is a cheaper and often

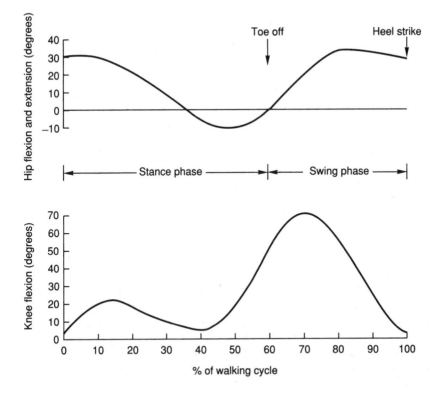

Fig. 9.6 Sagittal motion of hip and knee over one gait cycle (males).

technically easier method than the use of cinematic film or video recording.

It is evident that these methods show motion in only one plane – the sagittal – as described so far. Further, the distance over which body movement can be tracked is limited if a fixed camera is used. More sophisticated arrangements involve separate cameras to record movement in each plane and a provision for the cameras to track the moving subject in some way. The particular anatomical points that need to be seen to define the movement of interest can be specially marked to make them easy to follow on the recording.

Much data can be derived from such systems by considering separately the particular variables. The angles of the hip and knee can be plotted on the same graph, showing how each changes in different parts of the gait cycle (see Fig. 9.6). This figure shows clearly how the knee goes through two periods of flexion and never becomes fully extended in this example. The zero line is taken as the position in standing. Similarly, the instantaneous velocity of any body segment, say, the foot in Figure 9.5, can be plotted against position in the gait cycle. Many other variables, such as angular velocities and accelerations, can also be found.

A particularly widely used plot is that of one joint angle against

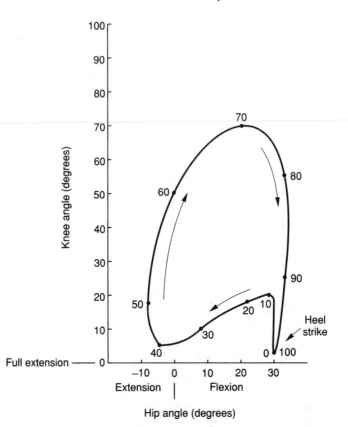

Fig. 9.7 Angle-angle diagram for hip against knee angles; percentages of cycle are shown on 'loop' (same data as Fig. 9.6).

another, the so called angle-angle diagrams. For example, the normal gait cycle produces a characteristic angle-angle diagram; see Figure 9.7, where the knee and hip angles are used. In disordered gaits, the diagrams for the two lower limbs will differ. Changes in gait pattern can conveniently be followed in a series of such plots taken over a period of time. The effects of surgery can also be monitored. Another method of producing these data directly is the use of electrogoniometers fitted to the hip and the knee so that the electrical output varies as the joints move during the walking cycle. In a suitable gait laboratory situation, the output from the potentiometers or strain gauges can be fed through suitable electronic analysis to produce an immediate angle-angle graph.

The force plate described in Chapter 3 provides information on sway, as noted, and it can also be used to give the pattern of pressure under the foot that occurs in walking, running, jumping etc.

Measurements of velocity and acceleration can be made for certain limited activities, such as walking in a straight line. A long paper tape with holes punched in it is attached to each heel, and, as the subject walks, the tape is drawn through a device that monitors and electronically stores the rate at which the holes move. From this, the velocity of lower limb motion can be calculated. Similar methods can be used for other segments.

Simple clinical recording of walking or running may be made on a suitable paper walkway, which coupled with timing of the walk, can give information of the velocity, step length etc.

Body segment accelerations can be measured by means of small accelerometers attached to the body, which have their electrical outputs continuously monitored. Simple accelerometers consist of a small mass of a few grams attached to a spring. Deflection of the spring is measured electrically when the small mass is accelerated. They usually only work in one direction so that analysis of complete movements involves the use of several accelerometers.

Electromyography, as mentioned in Chapter 6, allows the electrical changes due to muscle activity to be recorded. In a sense this is the only one of the measuring mechanisms that gives 'internal' information. By fixing electrodes close to individual muscles and muscle groups, either on the skin surface or with needle electrodes inserted into the muscle, it is possible to monitor muscle contraction. Up to a point, the magnitude can also be assessed. However, there are considerable technical difficulties associated with making accurate electromyographic recordings from muscles during activity.

It can be seen that several of these measuring methods need to be coupled electrically to some form of recording apparatus that is separate from the subject. Thus, the use of accelerometers and electrogoniometers, and electromyography, all need some electrical 'umbilical cord' connecting the recorder to the subject. This tends to inhibit the extent and nature of the activity to be assessed. Recently, small lightweight recorders have been developed, which can store the outputs over a period of time.

Various television/computer systems have been developed instantaneously to analyse and store body movement information. The use of two or three cameras allows the position in space of markers attached to the moving body segments to be automatically calculated at frequencies of 50 Hz or 60 Hz. Either reflective or 'active' markers are used. (Active markers are light-emitting diodes, which are made to flash sequentially.) From the changing positions of the markers, the relative position and movement of the body segments can be calculated by appropriate computer software.

While each of these systems produces valuable data on human movement, combining several measuring systems, such as taking electromyographic records of muscle activity while at the same time videoing the movement occurring, provides much more information. In laboratory and research settings this approach is being more and more widely used, since it is often considered that the value of a combined system is greater than the sum of its parts. The recent advances in electronic technology allow the enormous quantities of data produced by such systems to be processed and analysed. For clinical purposes, less technically demanding measurements are preferred but, as computing becomes cheaper, some quite complex systems are now available in the clinic.

GAIT

The word 'gait' is used synonymously with 'walking' in many contexts, but gait is considered to describe the manner of walking rather than the walking process itself. Thus walking may be considered a form of universal human locomotion performed in slightly different ways by different individuals – young, old, male, female etc. – who may be said to use different gaits (Whittle, 1991). From what has been described already, it can be seen that investigations of human movement have been largely concerned with walking; in fact, the historical development of biomechanics can be traced through studies of human walking (see Chapter 1).

Normal walking involves the alternate use of the two legs ('leg' is used for simplicity to mean 'lower limb') for support and propulsion, when at least one foot is always in contact with the ground. This distinguishes it from running, a clearly distinctive form of locomotion in which there is no contact with the ground during a part of the cycle. Of course, it is possible to walk backwards and sideways but these unusual gaits are not being considered.

A feature of normal walking on a level surface is the consistency of the repeated movements (cycles) of the activity. Of course, the movements are not perfectly identical but in a single individual they show remarkable consistency. This means that a single cycle can be used to describe the gait. While the general form of walking is universal, there are considerable variations of gait between individuals, which are not necessarily abnormal; it is difficult to define whether a particular gait is abnormal or simply a normal adaptation.

Description of gaits

The cycle time is the period between successive identical events. Usually the heel strike of one foot is taken as the event; the right heel strike is used in Figures 9.5–9.8. The position of the feet is used descriptively to define various points in the cycle. Each leg and foot goes through an identical cycle in which about 60% of the time is spent in contact with the ground – called the stance phase – and about 40% in moving forward – the swing phase. The whole cycle is called a 'stride' and is clearly formed of two 'steps', one by each foot. These events are represented in Figure 9.8, which shows the two periods of double support in which both feet are on the ground at the same time. These are separated by periods of stance on one leg while the other is in the swing phase. The gait cycle is often measured

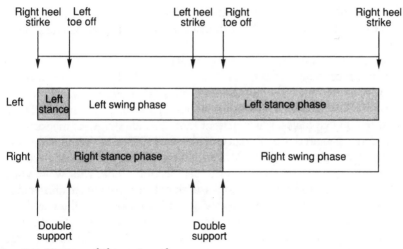

Fig. 9.8 Timing of the gait cycle.

clinically from a record of the footprints; much information can be gained from these foot placements (see Fig. 9.9):

1. *Stride length* is the distance between two successive placings of the same foot, e.g. two heel strikes, one directly in front of the other. In normal gait, the alternate *step lengths* (heel strike to opposite heel strike) are approximately equal. In all cases the stride length is the sum of the left and right step lengths.
2. *Step width* is the linear distance between the mid-heel points of the two feet. It is a line at right angles to the line of progression. It is also called the walking base.
3. *Foot angle* is the angle between the line of progression and a line through the long axis of the foot in the 'foot flat' portion of the cycle. It is usually a toe out angle.

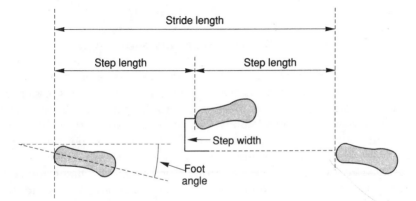

Fig. 9.9 Stride and step length.

Both of the latter two measurements reflect the lateral stability of the gait and tend to be increased in those with less efficient balance, such as the elderly.

Cadence is the number of steps or strides per unit time. Steps per second would be more correct, but steps per minute is often used. In both, it is clearly equal to twice the number of strides. The cadence varies with age and sex in normal adults, averaging about 118 steps per minute in females and about 113 in males. It is apparent that, if stride length is measured and the cadence counted, the velocity of the walker can be found. Consider a female with a stride length of 1.25 m and a cadence of exactly 120 steps per minute (conveniently 1 stride per second). She will walk with a velocity of 1.25 m s^{-1}. Similarly, measurement of the cadence and velocity, which are very simple clinical measurements to make (time the walk over a known distance and count the steps), allows the stride length to be calculated. The velocities of walking used by most people are remarkably consistent, being on average about 1.3 m s^{-1}, a little higher (1.37 m s^{-1}) for men and a little lower (1.23 m s^{-1}) for women (Smidt, 1990). Changes in walking speed occur all the time as walkers adjust their velocity to the conditions they meet: hurrying to keep an appointment or slowing to match the speed of a slower companion. While the velocity could be altered either by changing the stride length or the cadence, in reality it seems that both are changed. Increasing walking velocity is due to proportionally similar increases in both stride length and cadence until some maximum convenient stride length is reached, at which point cadence alone increases (Inman *et al.*, 1981). At a velocity of about 2.3 m s^{-1}, most adults change from walking to running in order to travel any faster. This occurs because the energy needed to walk above this speed is greater than the energy needed to run. It is persuasively argued that it is not only inefficient to walk much faster but actually impossible to walk with a normal gait beyond about 3 m s^{-1} (Alexander, 1992). Race walkers can achieve average speeds of around 4.4 m s^{-1}, but to do so they must use an unusual gait, which does not allow the centre of gravity to rise and fall so much.

Movements of the body segments during walking

Nearly all the body segments move in some way, some only to a trivial degree, during the gait cycle. Since the point of walking is progression in the forward direction, it seems sensible first to describe the motion of the centre of gravity of the whole body. The centre of gravity of the body, as discussed in Chapter 3, is a point that represents the mean position of the body mass. In the standing position it is situated centrally in the pelvis, approximately at the level of the second sacral vertebra. During forward walking, the legs move forwards and backwards, the arms swing and the trunk moves up and down and from side to side; consequently, the centre of gravity progresses forwards and at the same time moves up and down

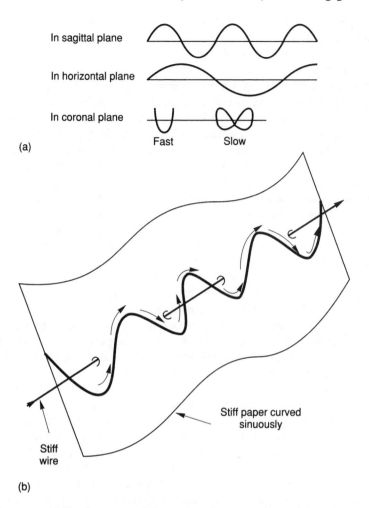

Fig. 9.10 (a) Displacement of the centre of gravity; (b) model to illustrate motion of the centre of gravity during walking.

and from side to side. Watching someone walking beside a horizontal line close to head height, say a wall or a hedge, makes the vertical motion that occurs become visible as the head appears to bob up and down at each step. This motion is sinusoidal and is about 50 mm in extent for adult males at normal walking speeds. The summits occur at the middle of the stance phase of each side; the lowest point occurs during double support when both feet are on the ground. The reason for this is the greater height of the body when supported on a vertical leg compared with when being supported by both legs at an angle to the vertical (see Fig. 9.10a).

The centre of gravity is also displaced in the horizontal plane, moving laterally to left and right as each alternate leg becomes weightbearing. It thus follows a smooth sinusoidal curve, but with only one oscillation per stride superimposed on the two vertical oscillations. Movement in this horizontal plane is also about 50 mm in extent for adult males (see Fig. 9.10a). The pathway that the centre of gravity takes in space is not easy to visualize or illustrate. A simple satisfactory model can be made by drawing a sinusoidal path on a piece of stiff paper and then bending the paper to conform with the lateral sinusoidal displacement, securing the position with a long stiff wire — a knitting needle will do — to represent the mean motion. This is illustrated in Figure 9.10b, but in reality the curves would be very much shallower than illustrated. As already noted, there would be a vertical and a lateral variation of only 5 cm in a stride of about 150 cm. Looking at such a model from the back or the front, it can be seen that the centre of gravity will oscillate in a coronal plane following a U-shape, rising and falling on each side and crossing the mid-line at its lowest. While this is reasonably true for fast walking, in slower walking the peak of the vertical displacement occurs before that of the lateral displacement, so that the path followed is a rather asymmetrical figure-of-eight (Inman *et al.*, 1981), as shown in Figure 9.10a.

As might be expected, the whole pelvis more or less follows the path of the centre of gravity, but tips slightly forward and backward and laterally. More significantly, it rotates about a vertical axis (around 12° in males), so that, as the left leg is advanced so the left side of the pelvis moves forward and vice versa. A similar but opposite rotation of somewhat less excursion occurs in the upper trunk and shoulder girdle association with arm swinging. Thus, as the left leg and left side of the pelvis are advanced, so also is the right shoulder, and the right arm swings forward.

In the lower limb, the hip flexes during the swing phase to bring the leg forward and extends during the stance phase, being at maximum just prior to toe off. The motion is illustrated in Figure 9.6. As can be seen, the hip joint is in some degree of flexion for about two-thirds of the walking cycle. In many descriptions of gait, the range of motion of the hip is combined with the slight forward and backward pelvic tilting noted above. The range of this pelvic motion increases with greater walking speeds but at normal speeds it seems to be around 5° in men and older women but rather more in young women (Hageman and Blanke, 1986).

The two flexion peaks that the knee goes through can be seen in Figure 9.6, the first early in the stance phase and the second, much larger, during the swing phases. It may be seen that the knee is already in quite marked flexion before the toe leaves the ground for the swing phase and has started to extend before the mid-point of the swing phase.

To some extent, the ankle joint follows the knee in that there are two phases of plantarflexion matching knee flexion and two of dorsiflexion matching knee extension. At heel strike, the ankle is in the neutral position (at right angles to the tibia) and is lowered into plantarflexion (by eccentric action of the dorsiflexors), bringing the foot flat on the ground. As the tibia moves forward over the stationary foot during stance, the ankle becomes steadily dorsiflexed until just after heel off. At this point, rapid plantarflexion occurs at the same time as the knee is flexing. At toe

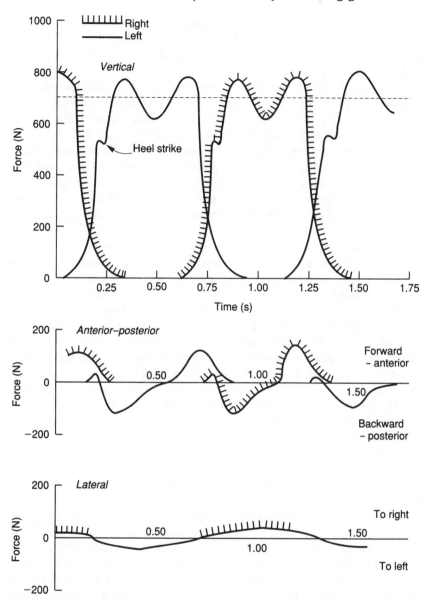

Fig. 9.11 Components of the ground reaction force as expressed by a typical force plate record.

off, the ankle dorsiflexes steadily as the leg swings forward to keep the toes clear of the ground, returning to the neutral position for the next heel strike.

The angle-angle diagram of Figure 9.7 illustrates the characteristic relationship between hip and knee angles. Diagrams relating knee angle to ankle angle, or any other pair of angles, can also be constructed. These tend to be highly consistent for an individual between steps and between the two sides. Discrepancy between the two sides is often the result of pathological changes, so that such graphs are useful as a clinical measurement of gait.

Since the centre of gravity is moving up and down it must be accelerated upwards so that at some point in the gait cycle a vertical force greater than the body weight must be exerted against the ground. Similarly at some other part of the cycle the descending mass of the body will exert a vertical force less than the body weight. These forces exerted by the feet on the ground can be registered on suitably arranged force plates, as described above and in Chapter 3. The typical output from a force plate shows a rapid force rise at heel strike followed by a smoother rise as the body is accelerated upwards with the hip moving into extension in the first part of the stance phase. As the body then starts to accelerate downwards the ground reaction force lessens to increase again as the body subsequently rises at toe off. Force plate records show this double peak of vertical force quite clearly as in Figure 9.11. The actual forces are critically dependent on the velocity of walking; faster walking means there is less time for the rise and fall of the body to occur so that the accelerations, and hence the forces, are larger. Although vertical forces are much the largest component, the actual forces are not only vertical but also have an anterior–posterior and a very small lateral component. This is to be expected since at heel strike the leg would be acting as a 'brake' to the forward motion, converting forward into upward motion. At toe off the leg pushes the body upwards and forwards. The lateral forces are comparatively small, being due to the need to shift the centre of gravity from side to side as described (see Fig. 9.11).

Muscle activity in gait

The muscles whose contractions produce walking have been extensively studied and the magnitude and sequence of their actions have been found to be highly variable. Not only is there great variability between individuals but the same person may utilize their muscles in a different way on different occasions; this is partly determined by differing walking speeds or varying degrees of fatigue. However, a typical pattern can be described, although it is by no means the only one possible. The following is based on Joseph (1964) and Inman et al. (1981). Much of the muscle activity occurs at the beginning and end of the stance phase, with rather less activity in mid-swing or mid-stance when most of the angular changes are taking place. Eccentric, isometric and concentric muscle activities all occur, sometimes sequentially in the same muscle or muscle group. Relatively little of this activity is concentric, which partly accounts for the great efficiency of walking in terms of metabolic energy (see Chapter 10).

At the start of the swing phase, the iliopsoas and tensor fasciae latae, which have just been stretched as the hip is extended at the end of stance, contract to initiate hip flexion. In some subjects, the adductors appear to contribute to hip flexion in the early swing stage. The anterior tibial group is active at toe off and continues contracting through the swing phase to keep the toe clear of the ground. They also work markedly at heel strike to lower the forefoot to the ground in a controlled way in the early part of stance.

Table 9.1 Summary of the muscle actions of walking

	Toe off	Foot off ground SWING PHASE	Heel strike	Foot on ground STANCE PHASE	Toe off
Iliopsoas and tensor fasciae latae		·:·::·.			
Tibialis anterior and toe extensors	·- : : : : : : : : : -		·::··		
Hamstring muscle group		·:·:·:·:·:·:·: :			
Sacrospinalis	·::·		·-·-·:·-·-		·:·:·
Gluteus medius and minimus				·:·:·:·:·:·:·:·:·:·:·.	
Gluteus maximus			·-·-·-·-·.		
Quadriceps	: ·		·:·:·:·:·:·. ·		·:·:·
Triceps surae			·:·:·:··::·:·:·. ·		

At the change from swing to the stance phase, several muscle groups become active. In the latter part of the swing phase, the hamstrings act to decelerate the swinging leg, continuing their activity into stance to extend the hip. (During faster walking they may also act minimally at toe off to help knee flexion.) Also, at the end of the swinging phase, the sacrospinalis exhibits a burst of activity to counteract the forward rotation of the pelvis (around a vertical axis) associated with the forward swing of the leg. This group contracts again at the end of the stance phase during toe off, as the body is being pushed upwards and forwards in order to prevent the trunk falling forwards. During the stance phase, the pelvis is supported on only one side so that the tendency to drop on the non-supported side is resisted by isometric contraction of the hip abductors, gluteus medius and gluteus minimus. This important action not only stabilizes the pelvis but also contributes to the rotation (around a vertical axis) of the pelvis as the opposite leg swings forward, with the muscles acting concentrically. Both the gluteus maximus and the quadriceps contract at the start of the stance phase, immediately after heel strike. The contribution of the gluteus maximus appears to be more marked in faster walking and acts to assist the hamstrings in extending the hip. The quadriceps acts eccentrically to restrict knee flexion. Later, at the end of the stance phase, as push off occurs, the quadriceps may contract again. The two heads of the gastrocnemius and soleus − the triceps surae − contract in the stance phase, starting early in the phase and finishing before the toe leaves the ground. Although this muscle action provides the propulsive force for walking, its action is almost isometric. A summary of these muscle actions is shown in Table 9.1. While this account of the muscles that are active in normal walking is valid, it must be repeated that there is considerable 'redundancy' in muscle able to produce a normal gait. Just because two gaits appear identical does not mean that exactly the same muscle action is occurring. Electromyographic investigations, on which the data for Table 9.1 are based, have repeatedly found variations.

Smooth, efficient walking

With legs nearly a metre long swinging through arcs over 40°, it may be wondered how the smooth sinusoidal path of the centre of gravity, as described above, is achieved and why it is of such small (≈50 mm) excursion. This is accounted for by several mechanisms that occur in normal walking and can be described as six separate elements. They are often called the six 'determinants' of gait. Although described separately they obviously act collectively.

1. Rotation of the pelvis: this occurs around a vertical axis and moves forwards the hip joint of the forward swinging leg. Thus, for any given stride length, less flexion and extension of the hip is needed because some of the stride length is due to pelvic motion. As a result of the smaller angles needed at the hip, there is less vertical movement of the trunk.
2. Pelvic tilt: as the hip of the stance leg rises, so the pelvis is allowed to tilt down on the other side, that of the swinging leg. This is controlled by the gluteus medius and minimus, as noted above, allowing the centre of gravity to remain lower than the stance phase hip. As the hip on the swing side is lower, it is necessary for the swinging leg to shorten to clear the ground. This is why the knee flexes and the ankle dorsiflexes.
3. Knee flexion of stance leg: this effectively shortens this leg in the middle of stance so that, as the leg passes from flexion to extension at the hip, it does not cause the hip to rise so much.
4. Ankle or heel mechanism: at heel strike the leg is effectively lengthened because the heel projects posteriorly; thus the hip is not lowered so much at the start of stance.

5. Forefoot mechanism: as the heel leaves the ground at the end of stance, the effective length of the leg is increased by the forefoot moving into plantarflexion. Thus determinants 3, 4 and 5 are all arranged to minimize the rise and fall of the hip of the stance side. Coupled with determinants 1 and 2, this ensures that the centre of gravity rises and falls in a smooth sinusoidal way through quite a small distance. It can be deduced from this, and from Figure 9.6, that, since there is no point in the gait cycle at which both the hip and the knee are fully extended at the same time, a walker's vertical height must be a little less than the standing height.

6. Lateral displacement: the side to side displacement of the pelvis is reduced by keeping the walking base narrow. The normal step width is only about 8 cm, so that very little lateral movement is needed to shift the centre of gravity over the stance leg. This is made possible by the valgus angulation at the knee, which allows the femoral heads to be separated by the width of the pelvis while the distal ends are close together, each being supported on a near vertical tibia.

What has been described above as 'normal' walking is a gait of around 1.3 m s^{-1} in adults but it is, of course, perfectly normal to walk at higher or lower velocities. As will be considered in Chapter 10, both changes are metabolically more expensive. In order to increase the speed of walking, the length of the stance phase is diminished and that of the swing phase increased. As noted earlier, both an increase in step length and cadence occur. As the stance phase shortens so does the period of double support until, at a velocity of around 2.3 m s^{-1}, it disappears altogether when the subject changes to a run. It should be understood that running is an entirely different gait, not a simple modification or progression of walking.

Development of walking

The development of independent, upright gait occurs in most children aged between 12 and 15 months. The timing seems to depend on neural maturation, making it frustratingly independent of parental encouragement! The importance of this milestone is linguistically recognized in the use of the word 'toddler' to describe children in their early walking stage. At first, the child walks with straight knees, planting the foot flat on the ground with no proper heel strike and usually with laterally rotated legs. This rapidly becomes more like the adult pattern but a wider base and a lack of arm swinging are evident until the child is about four years of age. By about the age of five, most children exhibit a normal adult gait pattern but, of course, the stride length is shorter and the cadence higher. This changes to more adult ranges as the child grows taller. While the average preferred velocities of free walking in children tend to be rather lower than in adults, they are quite close and even some two-year-olds overlap into the usual adult range of speeds.

In old age, the gait exhibits further changes. Some changes are due to disease, such as osteoarthritis or cerebrovascular dysfunction, which alter the gait pattern. When these are excluded, the gait of the elderly is little different from that of normal adults except that it is, on average, slowed down. There tends to be an increased walking base, either a greater step width or, more usually, increased toe out angle (Murray *et al.*, 1969). The stride length is also decreased, as is usually the cadence. A comparison between young and elderly women (Hageman and Blanke, 1986) also found that the younger women had a greater range of ankle motion and greater pelvic obliquity, i.e. rising more on one side. It is suggested (Murray *et al.*, 1969) that the nature of gait changes in the elderly is such as to improve security when there is less efficient balance; the balance loss in the elderly was noted in Chapter 3. Broadening the walking base, shortening the stride and decreasing the cadence all have this effect. Many of the other changes noted are a consequence of these. It has, however, been found that abnormally slow walking causes an unusual gait in the elderly (Gillis *et al.*, 1986). Again, it is suspected that this is due to more precarious balance.

The gait of otherwise normal subjects is affected by their mental state. While this is often recognized subjectively, with the association between feelings of well-being and a rapid energetic gait and the reverse, and is widely accepted there seems to be little objective evidence of changes in gait pattern. However, Sloman *et al.* (1982) found that a group of depressed patients walked with shorter stride lengths and with what the writers call a lifting motion rather than a propelling motion prior to toe off. They were unable to show that, as the depressed patients recovered, their gait became more normal. Thus, the question of whether depression caused the gait pattern changes, or whether a specific neuromuscular pattern is associated with susceptibility to depressive illness, remains unanswered.

This account of human gait biomechanics is necessarily brief and incomplete. An excellent introduction to gait analysis can be found in Michael Whittle's book (1991) and the thorough classical work of Inman *et al.* (1981) and Murray *et al.* (1964) are invaluable.

RUNNING

Running is not a simple progression of walking; it is a quite distinct gait with different characteristics. It is noticeable that the change from walking to running is made abruptly, one stride is a walk, the next a run. The distinction, as already noted, is that in running there are phases when neither foot is in contact with the ground. It is a series of 'leaps' and inevitably involves much greater knee flexion, both of the supporting and the swinging leg, than does walking. In both walking and running, the body rises and falls at each step, more so in running. It has just been shown how adjustments are made in walking to limit the amount of rise and fall of the body, which are the first five 'determinants' of gait. Even so, the centre of gravity is still required to rise and fall some 50 mm in an averagely tall male subject. At heel strike, the centre of gravity is moved upwards and forwards but it loses velocity as it does so. At the mid-point of stance, it descends towards the opposite heel strike, gaining velocity as it does so. Thus, provided the legs remain nearly straight, as they do in walking, there is a constant interchange between kinetic energy (the velocity of movement) and potential energy (the height of the centre of gravity), with little loss as one form is exchanged for the other. It is like the changes that occur as a pendulum swings to and fro. These mechanisms, which make walking so efficient in terms of energy used per metre travelled, are not utilized in running. Yet running, although not as efficient as the preferred walking pace of 1.3–1.4 m s^{-1} or so, is efficient compared with fast or very slow walking. How can this be achieved? The answer seems to be that connective tissue elasticity (see Chapter 2) is utilized to return energy to the system; in running the legs are used more like springs than rigid supports.

During running, the heel usually (but not always) hits the ground first, but contact is rapidly moved forward on to the metatarsophalangeal joints. As this weight transference is proceeding, the triceps surae and quadriceps are lengthening a little to allow bending of the knee and dorsiflexion of the foot. Subsequently, the centre of gravity passes forward of this supporting leg, at which point the knee extends and the ankle plantarflexes by means of quadriceps and triceps surae contraction, to thrust the rest of the body upwards and forwards. The supporting foot then leaves the ground. During the whole of this supporting and propelling action, the opposite leg has been off the ground with the knee markedly flexed, being moved rapidly forward by flexion at the hip joint. As the propelling foot leaves the ground, the knee of the other side rapidly extends to position the foot for the next heel strike. At this point, the body is moving through the air ('flying') with neither foot on the ground. Of course, running at different speeds produces different gaits. Sprinting involves longer strides, with more knee flexion of the swinging leg, a greater forward lean and more vigorous arm movements compared with a jogging-type gait. In some running gaits, the forefoot makes first contact with the ground instead of the heel. This often occurs when running on hard surfaces.

It was stated above that, in the early part of the stance phase of running, the quadriceps and triceps surae elongate but this was a simplification. Certainly these and other muscles have been shown by electromyography to be active in running, but much of the joint movement observed is found to be due to the stretching of their tendons. The elasticity of collagen tissue was considered in Chapter 2 and it was noted that tendons can be stretched up to 8% of their length and recoil elastically. It has been calculated that the tendo calcaneus is stretched by some 6% in running (Alexander, 1992). Since the arch of the foot is flattened as the ankle moves into dorsiflexion, the supporting ligaments are also stretched. In order that the tendons are stretched, their muscles must be in contraction but this can be isometric or nearly so. As explained in Chapter 5, isometric and, even more so, eccentric contractions are metabolically more efficient than concentric contractions. Thus, by using the tendons and ligaments as springs, much of the energy used is returned to help accelerate the body upwards. It has been calculated from force plate data that about a third of the total energy of each step is stored and returned by the tendo calcaneus and about one-sixth by the arch of the foot (Alexander, 1992). With a similar effect in the quadriceps tendon, less than half the energy has to be provided by muscles lengthening and shortening.

Running speeds vary from about $2.5 \, \text{m s}^{-1}$ up to about $10 \, \text{m s}^{-1}$ for good sprinters over 100 m or less. It is well recognized that the higher speeds can only be maintained over short distances, in which most of the muscular energy comes from anaerobic processes. Over a longer distance, speed is limited by the capacity of the cardiovascular system, as described in Chapter 10. Thus, the appropriate world record speeds for the distances shown in Table 9.2 can be seen to decrease sharply in the longer races.

Table 9.2 Approximate speeds of men's world records

Distance (m)	Speed (m s^{-1})
100	10.2
1000	7.6
1500	6.7
10 000	6.1

Such speeds are rather low compared with some animals; horses racing over one mile (1600 m) can better $16 \, \text{m s}^{-1}$. In sprinting, all the energy is directed to increasing speed at the expense of economy. Thus, there is much greater pelvic motion to give a greater stride length. Stride lengths over 2 m at a cadence of around 150 per minute are seen in male sprinting (Dyson, 1968) with vigorous reciprocal movements of arms and shoulders. (These latter allow the rapid pelvic rotation about a vertical axis needed for long striding by providing a reaction force and greater stretch in the rotator muscles.) One factor limiting the velocity of leg movements – hence of the sprint – is the moment of inertia of the leg. As discussed earlier, the angular momentum is the product of the moment of inertia and the angular velocity. Thus, in order to increase the angular velocity of the forward swinging leg, it is necessary to reduce the moment of inertia by bringing the centre of gravity of the lower limb closer to the axis of motion, the hip. This allows the limb to be swung forward more rapidly. It is notable that many fast running animals (horses, deer etc.), have the main mass of the limbs – the bulk of the muscles – close to the body, while the rest of each limb is long and slender. Furthermore, bending the knee in sprinting reduces air resistance, since the foot is not swung forwards at quite such a high velocity. It will be recalled from Chapter 6 that velocity is the important factor (drag rises with the square of the velocity) and it has been calculated from wind tunnel experiments that air resistance accounts for some 13% of the drag during sprinting (Alexander, 1992).

In starting a sprint, it is necessary to accelerate the body; sprinters start from a forward leaning position so that the straightening lower limb will drive the centre of gravity both upwards and forwards. Film recording has shown that acceleration over the first few strides can approximate to that due to gravity, i.e. nearly $10 \, \mathrm{m \, s^{-1}}$, in some sprinters. (This is, of course, well in excess of the much advertised acceleration of sports cars, unless they are being driven over a cliff!) As a sprinter's speed increases, so the force that can be exerted to produce forward acceleration decreases and a more upright posture is adopted. For the downward and backward force of the legs to produce a forward acceleration, it must necessarily be opposed by the ground reaction force and hence there must be sufficient friction between the shoe and the ground, as considered in Chapter 6. Since the reaction force and the frictional force are nearly identical – the acceleration due to gravity pressing the shoe on the ground and the horizontal acceleration are both about $10 \, \mathrm{m \, s^{-1}}$ – then their ratio is 1, so that the coefficient of friction is at least 1. In fact, tests of rubber soled running soles on various surfaces give values of 1.0–1.5 for the coefficient of friction (see also Chapter 6; table 6.1 shows rubber on concrete as 1.2). It is difficult to ascertain the precise pattern of muscular activity in running but it would appear to involve the muscle groups that would be expected from their known actions and contribution to walking, i.e. the principal flexors and extensors of the lower limbs, with additional activity in the trunk and arm musculature. While walking is performed with surprisingly little muscle activity, with that which does occur appearing later and finishing sooner than might be expected, running involves much more extensive and prolonged activity. Important groups of muscles not previously mentioned are those that stabilize the foot and the toes – principally the intrinsic foot muscles and long flexors of the toes – to allow them to act in both support and propulsion when the foot is on the ground. This occurs in both walking and running but more markedly in the latter since the forces are so much greater. The flexor hallucis longus appears to make a particularly significant contribution in stabilizing the metatarsophalangeal joint of the big toe and pressing the big toe on the ground at the final part of toe off. In both walking and running, heel strike occurs nearer the lateral edge of the heel, and the centre of pressure on the foot moves forward and medially during stance to the big toe at toe off.

CLIMBING STAIRS

Climbing stairs involves considerable modification of gait. The weight is first transferred on to one leg to allow the other to be flexed at the hip and the knee, dorsiflexed at the ankle, and swung on to the step above. To gain sufficient height for the free foot to top this step — which for most steps is about 15 cm — not only are the hip and knee markedly flexed but the pelvis on that side is not allowed to sag and may even be elevated by the action of the opposite weightbearing limb hip abductors. Importantly, the plantarflexors of this leg raise the heel, lifting the whole body upwards. Simultaneously, the whole foot (sometimes the forefoot only) contacts the step above, and extension of the hip and knee of this forward leg, due to contraction of the hip extensors and quadriceps, aids elevation of the whole body. The forward lean of the trunk shifts the centre of gravity over this forward leg so that the rearward leg is now non-weightbearing, and, at toe off, flexes at the hip and the knee and dorsiflexes to clear the step, continuing on to the next step above to repeat the cycle. Descending is not a simple reversal because the centre of gravity must be maintained over one leg, which is flexing at the knee — strong eccentric contraction of the quadriceps — while the other is lowered to the step below. This lower forward limb contacts the step with the forefoot, allowing the body weight to be transferred forwards and downwards as the foot dorsiflexes and the knee flexes to continue the cycle, with the other leg moving forwards to the succeeding step. It may be noted that, in descending, the body weight is lowered entirely on one lower limb, most of the energy being absorbed by the quadriceps working eccentrically. When ascending, the body weight is elevated both by the knee and the hip extensors of one leg and by the triceps surae of the opposite leg as the body is accelerated upward by the rearmost leg. This accounts for the finding that some patients with knee injuries suffer pain on descending but not on climbing stairs. Not surprisingly, going upstairs uses more metabolic energy but coming down causes more muscular discomfort. Anyone climbing a tall spiral staircase — like the 311 steps of the Monument in London or the 698 steps of the Washington Monument — will recognize that going up causes breathlessness and coming down makes the legs ache!

JUMPING

Some consideration was given earlier in this chapter to a standing jump. It will be known that even the most athletic of people can only jump about 1.5 m by using this method, yet a normal high jumper using a run up can clear over 2 m (the men's high jump record is about 2.44 m). Since the take-off for such high jumps is from one leg only, it may be wondered why much greater height can be achieved when compared with the squat-type jump that uses both legs. The answer is that some of the kinetic energy generated during the run up is used to gain height by being converted to potential energy. At the end of the run up, one of the jumper's feet is planted down well in front of the moving body with the knee almost straight. As the centre of gravity moves further forwards, the knee bends somewhat and then rapidly extends, throwing the jumper upwards. There is still enough forward motion to carry the athlete over the bar. The forward leg acts rather like a springy pole, storing the kinetic energy of the run up and returning it as vertical movement, in the same way that a pole vaulter uses the energy of the run up to bend the pole and the elastic recovery of the pole to gain height. (Of course, the pole is much more efficient, so that pole vaulters can clear between 5 and 6 m.) Some data from Alexander (1992) from a filmed men's high jump competition shows that about half the kinetic energy of the jump is converted to potential energy of height. Just prior to take off they ran at 6.7 m s^{-1} and their mass was 76 kg (all mean figures). Thus, their kinetic energy at $\frac{1}{2}mv^2 = \frac{1}{2} \times 76 \times 6.7^2$, which is 1705.8 joules. While crossing the bar, their speed was 4.2 m s^{-1}, so that they still had $\frac{1}{2} \times 76 \times 4.2^2 = 670.3$ joules of kinetic energy. Thus 1035.5 joules had been used to gain height. Their centres of gravity rose from a mean of 0.91 m to 2.1 m, i.e. 1.19 m so the potential energy gained equalled 'm g h' or $76 \times 9.81 \times 1.19 = 887.2$ joules. The discrepancy of 148 joules can probably be accounted for by some rotary motion imparted to the body and heat losses (Alexander, 1992).

The concept of exchanges between kinetic and potential energies is widely exploited in human movement. Pendular motion, in which the height of the bob at each extreme – the potential energy – is exchanged for motion – kinetic energy – at each swing, is found in many body movements, in the description of gait given above, for example. In all such systems, some energy will be lost at each exchange – at each oscillation – so that a little energy needs to be added at each swing to maintain a constant amplitude, otherwise it diminishes. In all kinds of repetitive activities in which body segments move in a regular reciprocal pattern, considerable conservation of energy is achieved if the motion occurs at the 'natural' frequency, i.e. the frequency appropriate to the length of the particular 'pendulum' involved. The potential energy does not need to be gravitational in the form of height but can be the elasticity of tissues. These mechanisms operate not only in walking and running, as considered, but in any reciprocating activity (rowing, sawing wood, cycling etc.). In these situations, it is not only the mass of the body segments that is involved but also the mechanical moving parts (saw, cycle). Consider two men loading heavy sacks onto a high truck. The sacks are swung between them in a pendular manner two or three times, so that the kinetic energy of the swing can be used as they throw the sacks upwards; in a way the sacks are made to take a 'running jump'.

In long jumping, the forward leg is set down and the knee flexes then extends as in high jumping, but the leg is not set down so far in front of the body as in high jumpers and the run up is faster. These two differences enable the jumper to travel a greater horizontal distance. It may be wondered why high jumpers do not run up at their maximum speed; the 6.7 m s^{-1} quoted above is clearly below the 9.5 m s^{-1} or so that most good athletes might achieve. This seems to be due to the need for the foot to remain at one point on the ground to achieve the optimum acceleration time (Alexander, 1992).

CONTROL OF MOVEMENT

All movement is initiated and controlled through the neuromuscular system. it is evident that such control needs to be extremely complex. Even the simplest movement involves precisely executed muscle contractions – precise in both force and timing – as well as adjustments to adjacent body segments and body posture. It has been pointed out (Butler and Major, 1992) that in standing, for example, movement between any pair of body segments (thigh and pelvis or leg and thigh etc.) requires a response from at least two other joints. In all situations, just to maintain a static posture requires a continuous inflow of sensory (proprioceptive, cutaneous and visual) information, coupled to precise muscular adjustments; this is partly described in Chapter 3. Increasing the activity, such as adding the leg and arm movement in walking as discussed above, enormously increases the adjustments needed.

It is neither possible nor appropriate adequately to describe or explain motor control in this book. Readers should consult suitable neurophysiological texts. The basis of movement is considered to be reflex, that is, information is received and processed, and then stimulates the effector organs, the muscles. In the nervous system, afferent information is provided by numerous sensory systems, as indicated in Table 9.3.

For the control of muscular activity, the muscle spindles are of particular significance, since they are not only able to signal muscle stretch but can be themselves adjusted to signal at differing degrees of stretch. The input from these various sources (Table 9.3) is not discrete but integrated into the central nervous system to provide specific information on body motion. Thus, for example, head movement, detected by the vestibular apparatus and the eyes, is coupled with input from joint receptors in the neck to determine whether the trunk is in motion or only the head. The effector organs, the muscles, are under nervous control from the anterior horn cells via motor units in the muscle, as noted in Chapter 4. As described, the tension developed in muscle depends on the number of motor units being stimulated and the rate at which they fire. The timing of muscle contraction also depends on the times at which the nerve impulses occur.

The connector neurones between the afferent and efferent pathways are found in the central nervous system. All movement is considered to be based upon reflex activities, which are initially the inherited inborn patterns of movement. Upon these are built the learned motor skills by both maturation of the nervous system and motor learning from the repeated practice of particular motor patterns. Many simple motor reflexes are recognized as stereotyped responses, which can often easily be seen in

Table 9.3 Sensory sources providing information for movement

Group	Name	Location	Stimulated by
Proprioceptors	Muscle spindles	Muscles	Stretch of muscles
	Golgi tendon organs	Tendons	Stretch of tendons
	Type I joint receptors	Capsule of joint (superficial layers)	Position of joint
	Type II joint receptors	Capsule of joint (deep layers)	Movement of joint
	Type III joint receptors	Joint ligaments	Stretch of ligament
	Hair cells of vestibular apparatus	Inner ear	Head position and movement
Exteroceptors			
Cutaneous sense organs	Mechanoreceptors	Skin	Pressure
Special sense organs	Visual receptors	Eyes	Visual information

the newborn, for example, stretch reflexes, withdrawal reflexes, righting reflexes and many others. During development, controlled movement appears, as higher centres in the nervous system become able to direct movement and inhibit some of the automatic, but unwanted, reflex responses.

Even the simplest motor reflex requires considerable co-ordination between the participating muscles − relaxation of antagonists, appropriately timed contraction of synergists and stabilizers, and so forth − all of which is integrated in the spinal cord and brain centres to produce automatic movement. This aspect is entirely unconscious. It is all based on continuous information about the position and movement of the body and its segments. Much of this information becomes available to centres in the brain, which are able to provide conscious recognition where it can be interpreted and where signals can be sent to modify those movements, hence effecting voluntary control. Particular aspects of movement are involved in different parts of the central nervous system. This has been deduced from the consequences of disease affecting localized areas. Thus, the motor area of the cerebral cortex in front of the central sulcus is concerned with volitional movement, on the opposite side of the body, through neurones grouped as the corticospinal system. Similar groupings involving the balance mechanism, designated the vestibulospinal system, are involved in the maintenance of the upright position.

Learning a skilled movement involves the acquisition of a particular facility in performing some movement. It can refer to a skill acquired by children as they mature, which might be regarded as a normal ability in adults – such as being able to stand on one leg – as well as a skill not normally found, such as being able to balance on a tightrope. Motor skills are learned largely by attempted repetition. It is characteristic of skilled movement that it is economical of muscle activity. The learning of a new motor skill seems to involve the inhibition of unwanted muscular actions. Exactly how such learning might occur in the nervous system is not known, but it is presumed that particular neural circuits – chains of neurones – become habituated and hence utilized when the appropriate stimulus occurs.

The contribution of mechanical factors such as the exchanges between kinetic and potential energy in the control of walking has already been noted. Such factors as the mass of the limb segments, the position of the centres of gravity, and the way that muscles and tendons can act as springs, have all been considered and will all contribute to the control of limb motion in any rhythmical activity. Such influences are considered as the biodynamic theory of limb motion (Beheshti, 1994), sometimes regarded as an alternative to the neurophysiological theory, which emphasizes activity in the central nervous system.

The acquisition of new motor skills and the re-education of those that have been lost as a result of disease or injury are central to the practice of physiotherapy. The teaching of motor skills for therapeutic purposes is dealt with in many extensive texts. Learning skills can also be considered from other theoretical perspectives, for example, broken down into three steps of perception, decision and movement organization as operations in the central nervous system (Marteniuk, 1979).

The importance of the higher centres of the brain in acquiring motor skills has not yet been emphasized. Apart from the obvious need for voluntary intention and determination repeatedly to practise the movements, there appears to be a considerable involvement of mental imagery. Mental practice or symbolic rehearsal of a skilled physical activity has been found to be beneficial in many sports and to have considerable therapeutic potential (Harrison and Jackson, 1994)

Discussion of human motion in this chapter has been centred upon normal movement. A full understanding of the normal is needed prior to consideration of disordered movement. It can be seen that any disruption of the physical structure – loss of motion at a joint or alteration of bone alignment – will lead to one kind of movement disorder, while some loss of the control system, either sensory input or motor output, will cause a different kind of disorder. Some of the methods of analysis can contribute to the diagnosis and tracking of the development of movement disorders, in which an understanding of the complexities of normal human motion is an essential foundation for diagnosis and therapy.

10. *Energy, efficiency and endurance in human movement*

Human movement results from muscular activity, which has been discussed in Chapter 4 to some extent, but it is evident that different kinds of movement involve, and are limited by, different mechanisms. A slow muscle contraction found in, say, heavy weightlifting or the isometric contraction in supporting a heavy weight for a few seconds, involves great muscle force being exerted; this is often referred to as 'strength'. The maximum weight that can be lifted is limited by the force capacity of the muscle tissue involved for any given circumstance. The more muscle tissue there is available, the more force can be exerted. This is seen in competitive weightlifting in that heavier men, having more muscle mass, can lift heavier weights. If the activity depends on movement, then muscle shortening must occur. The work done by the muscle depends on the force it exerts multiplied by the distance it shortens;

$$\text{work (or energy)} = \text{force} \times \text{distance}$$

A muscle contracting isometrically does no external mechanical work; it acts externally like a solid object providing support. There are, of course, energy exchanges going on within the muscle: the cross-bridging described in Chapter 4. When the muscle shortens through some distance, then external mechanical work is done and the rate at which this work is done (the power) will depend on the time it takes to shorten through the given distance. Formally:

$$\frac{\text{force (N)} \times \text{distance (m)}}{\text{time (s)}} = \frac{\text{work (energy) (J)}}{\text{time (s)}} = \text{power (W)}$$

as described in Chapter 1.

In order to shorten at higher and higher rates, the muscle can exert less and less external force, as shown in Figure 4.3, until, at the maximum rate of shortening, it can exert no external force at all. The energy is all used in causing the muscle itself to shorten while overcoming internal resistances, so that there is no external force exerted and hence no power. If the output power is plotted against the rate of shortening, as illustrated in Figure 10.1, it can be seen that the maximum power – the greatest rate of work – that the muscle can achieve will occur between the extremes of an isometric contraction and an isotonic contraction performed at the maximum rate. Thus, the activity is most efficient where moderate force is exerted at moderate rates of shortening. This is important in circumstances

Basic Biomechanics Explained

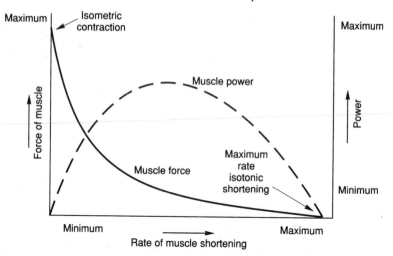

Fig. 10.1 Muscle force and power plotted against rate of shortening.

in which maximum efficiency is the critical factor. Long distance cycle racers, for example, use gears to keep their rate of leg movement roughly constant when travelling up and down hills. Of course, efficiency is not always the main concern, so that, in a sprint race, the muscle may be shortening at higher rates to give faster limb movement. The rate at which the muscle can work is, of course, limited by the rate at which chemical energy in the muscle can cause cross-bridges to form and separate, as described in Chapter 4. In common with other cells, muscle uses the hydrolysis of adenosine triphosphate (ATP) to provide energy for the mechanical changes. The resulting separation of a phosphate molecule and formation of adenosine diphosphate (ADP) in large amounts is diminished in contracting muscle by the presence of quantities of phosphocreatine; this is able to combine with ADP to recreate ATP and release creatine. While this, and some other reactions, are able to maintain suitable levels of ATP in contracting muscle for a short time, ultimately the rapid use of ATP in the vigorously contracting muscle far outstrips its synthesis. Synthesis of ATP is effected by the anaerobic breakdown of glucose to pyruvate, but each glucose molecule forms only two molecules of ATP. Further breakdown of the pyruvate in the tricarboxylic acid cycle (TCA, Krebs or citric acid cycle) of the mitochondria, in which it is oxidized, will lead to the formation of 36 molecules of ATP per glucose molecule. Thus, the aerobic production of ATP is of most consequence; for muscle contractions to be sustained their energy use must not outstrip the rate of oxygenation, as described below. It would therefore be expected that the power that muscles can generate would be high during the first few seconds but much less for sustained activity. This is common experience and is seen in the different running velocities for sprinters and middle distance runners described in Chapter 9.

Over the first few seconds of contraction, the muscle energy comes almost entirely from ATP and the creatine phosphate already present in the muscle. The aerobic processes are stimulated and their activity increases rapidly over the initial few seconds, then more slowly. If the exercise is moderate, the contractions may be maintained aerobically but, if the exercise is severe, glycolysis also starts to occur after the first few seconds.

The power that can be generated during short bursts of activity (for about 6 s) has been measured from subjects using bicycle ergometers. (This actually only measures leg muscle activity, but that is a considerable proportion of body muscle.) It was found that, as might be expected, international sprinters were able to generate more total power (over 1000 W) and more power per kilogram of body weight than recreational runners. Women were found to generate rather less power, both total and as a function of body weight, than (athletically) equivalent men. However, both international and recreational endurance male runners had similar power outputs at about 12 watts per kilogram ($W kg^{-1}$), with female recreational runners producing rather less at about $10 W kg^{-1}$. The idea that power over a few seconds is limited by the nature of muscle contraction has already been seen in Figures 4.3 and 10.1, which show the force–velocity curve for a concentric muscle contraction. This type of curve is characteristic of all muscle tissue and all points on it satisfy an equation (called Hill's equation, from the famous muscle physiologist A. V. Hill). This shows that the velocity (v) equals the maximum muscle force (F_{max}) minus the actual force (F_{act}) multiplied by a constant (b) and divided by the actual force plus a constant (a). Thus:

$$V = \frac{(F_{max} - F_{act}) \times b}{(F_{act} + a)}$$

Note that 'a' is a constant with the dimensions of force while 'b' has the dimensions of velocity. This indicates that for all muscle tissue there is a fixed limit to the velocity of shortening and the force of contraction. Thus, the way in which limb velocity in the human body can be increased is by means of a suitable leverage system, as discussed in Chapter 5. Similarly, the only method of increasing force is by using larger muscles – more muscle tissue – as noted under 'muscle architecture' in Chapter 4.

For muscle activity to be continued for a long period, it must be maintained at relatively low power. The ability to maintain activity is called endurance and is limited in the muscles by what is called muscle fatigue, but, when large muscle masses are involved, it is limited by the ability of the cardiovascular system to deliver oxygen to and remove carbon dioxide from the working muscles. The discussion of fatigue in Chapter 4 is of relevance. Thus, if a large proportion of the body musculature is involved, it is the cardiovascular and respiratory systems that determine the limits of activity and hence dictate the rate of that activity, for instance in distance running. If only a small proportion of the muscle mass is working, the activity may be continued for very long periods with many repetitions, like walking for example, or in many working situations in which low force repetitive movements are required. Such activity is often limited by fatigue in the muscle coupled with other aspects of fatigue in the central nervous system, see Chapter 4.

The concept that has been discussed above is summarized in Table 10.1, with the important proviso that the categories described should not be regarded as mutually exclusive, as much exercise activity overlaps several categories. It is not, of course, being suggested that sprinters do not become breathless or long distance racing cyclists do not use high muscle power; it is simply a framework on which the generalized relative features of different kinds of activity can be fitted. The distinctions are seen quite clearly at the higher levels of athletic sports in which different body types dominate, as described in Chapter 3. Thus, weightlifters and discus throwers are heavily muscled and capable of a single explosive muscle contraction, whereas sprinters are able to produce high muscle power and endurance runners are able to provide high levels of tissue oxygenation for long periods. This latter ability needs not only efficient cardiovascular and respiratory systems but also the capability to lose excess heat easily and rapidly, which occurs more readily in those of tall slender build (also noted in Chapter 3). A distinction needs to be made between relative and absolute muscle power or muscle force. Heavier weightlifters are able to lift heavier weights because they have greater absolute strength but, if the strength (muscle force) is expressed as a function of the body weight – in newtons per kilogram – they may be lifting less than a lighter man (see Fig. 4.9b). The same applies to power measurements, which can be expressed as watts per kilogram.

Table 10.1 Categories of muscular performance

Force and rate	No. muscle contractions	Examples	Limiting factor
Large force, low rate	Single, slow or isometric	Lifting weights	Quantity, quality and type of muscle tissue
Large force, high rate (power)	Several	Sprinting Jumping	As above
Low force, low rate	Large number of muscle contractions involving a large proportion of total muscle mass	Distance running, cycle racing	Ability of cardiovascular and respiratory systems
Low force, low rate	Large number of muscle contractions involving a small proportion of the total muscle mass	Picking fruit, typing	Fatigue of muscles

GENERAL PHYSIOLOGICAL CHANGES THAT OCCUR IN EXERCISE

As just noted, there are significant physiological changes that occur in the body to maintain long, continued muscular exertion, which involves the cardiovascular and respiratory systems. These will only be outlined; for a detailed elucidation, the appropriate physiology texts should be consulted.

When muscle contraction occurs, ATP and phosphocreatine are used and ADP and creatine are formed. These processes must be reversed and ATP be reformed for continued muscle function. Some ATP is produced by glycolysis in the muscle and much more by oxidation of carbon compounds in the TCA cycle in the mitochondria. Thus, for continuing muscle contraction to occur, a supply of glucose (forming pyruvate), fatty acids, ketone bodies and oxygen are needed, as well as the removal of carbon dioxide to allow the TCA cycle to operate. While some of these compounds are already stored in the muscle – notably, muscle glycogen and triglyceride – the supply must be rapidly renewed via the circulating blood. This is summarized in Table 10.2.

These chemical processes and mechanical changes also produce a good deal of heat, which has to be transferred away from the muscle tissue. This need for transport to (oxygen and carbon compounds) and from (carbon dioxide, lactate and heat) the muscle is achieved by increased blood flow due to dilatation of muscle capillaries. This is thought to be induced by changes in the local blood chemistry, notably the increased acidity due to carbon dioxide and lactate. The very activity of repeated muscular contraction and relaxation leads to varying pressure on the soft-walled veins, which mechanically increases blood flow. This effective lowering of the peripheral resistance is coupled with an increased cardiac output (both heart rate and stroke volume) to raise the blood flow. There may also be some increase in blood pressure. The extent of the increase in cardiac output naturally depends on the extent of the exercise, both the severity and the mass of muscle tissue involved. At rest, the adult cardiac output might be about five litres per minute. In vigorous exercise this could rise to 25 litres per minute. More usually, moderate exercise would raise the cardiac output to, perhaps, three times its resting value. At the same time, the principal reason for increased intramuscular blood flow, the exchange of oxygen and carbon dioxide between erythrocytes and muscle tissue, is greatly increased. This occurs because the raised acidity and temperature allow the erythrocyte haemoglobin to exchange a greater proportion of its transported gases. Consequential to the increased systemic blood flow is an identical increase in pulmonary blood flow and an associated increase in the rate and depth of respiration. This allows the increased gas exchange in the lungs to keep pace with the oxygen needs and excretion of carbon dioxide.

The heat generated by the working muscles is at first dissipated throughout other tissues and, as the general body temperature starts to rise, appropriate heat loss mechanisms are brought into play to maintain a

Table 10.2 Synthesis of ATP in muscle

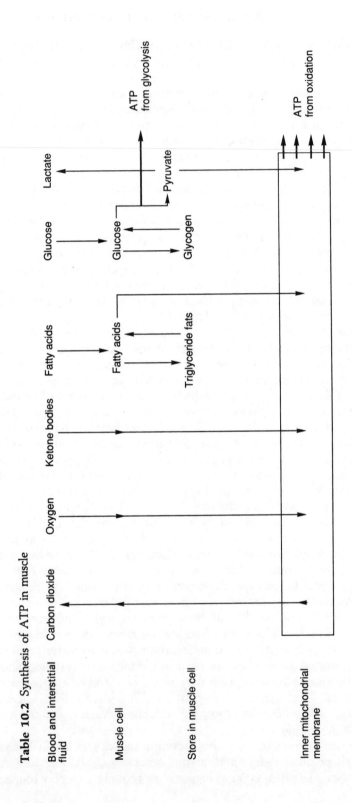

constant temperature. A small rise of local tissue temperature does seem to be beneficial for muscle activity, in that it allows greater oxygen dissociation, more rapid enzymic action and, perhaps, more rapid flow (because of the lowered viscosity). In vigorous exercise, general body temperature may rise a degree or so but eventually marked cutaneous vasodilation allows a more rapid heat loss through the skin at low environmental temperatures. When the outside temperature is high, sweating is needed to allow evaporation of water from the skin surface to provide cooling and thus attain, and maintain, heat balance.

Numerous further changes occur in body systems to facilitate prolonged muscular exercise. For instance, while the muscle blood flow is enhanced, that in the excretory and digestive organs is decreased due to vasoconstriction. Such a mechanism helps to keep a more nearly constant peripheral resistance and so maintain the arterial blood pressure. Furthermore, the blood glucose used by muscle is replaced by that from glycogen stored in the liver. Some of the lactate formed in the muscles when glucose is broken down is transported to the liver, where it is reconverted to glucose and returned via the circulating blood by a mechanism known as the Cori cycle. The quantity of circulating erythrocytes and the blood volume can be raised by contraction of the spleen during exercise.

The control of all these mechanisms is extremely complex. Ultimately, control is effected by both nervous and hormonal mechanisms, which are firmly integrated. In general, the sympathetic division of the autonomic nervous system promotes voluntary muscle activity in association with adrenaline and noradrenaline. Anticipation of vigorous exercise can lead to an increased heart rate and other appropriate physiological adjustments prior to the actual onset of the exercise; this illustrates the role of higher centres in the control systems.

AEROBIC AND ANAEROBIC MUSCLE ACTIVITY

It has been seen that there are basically three sources of ATP replacement as muscle tissue contracts:

1. ATP and phosphocreatine stored in the muscle itself;
2. The breakdown of glucose to pyruvate (glycolysis), the glucose being derived from both muscle glycogen and the circulating blood;
3. The operation of the TCA cycle to re-form ATP.

The last source requires oxygen whereas the first two do not (see Table 10.2). Explosive muscle contractions lasting only a few seconds are therefore fuelled from the stored creatine and ATP, whereas muscles continuing to exercise for more than 8–10 s draw more of their energy from glycolysis and, as the length of time increases, more energy replacement must come from the operation of the TCA cycle. Since oxygen is essential for the latter, it is called 'aerobic' whereas the other two sources are 'anaerobic'. Only limited amounts of ATP, creatine phosphate and glucose are stored in the muscle or replaced via the Cori cycle, so high rates of energy expenditure are only possible for a short time until these stores are depleted. After this period, the rate of muscle energy expenditure is limited by oxygen delivery etc., and is therefore at a lower level. If vigorous exercise is undertaken for a short time, the physiological changes involved in delivering oxygen to the tissues (increased respiration and heart rate etc.) continue for some time after the exercise is completed. This is to replace ATP and creatine phosphate stores and is reasonably described as 'oxygen debt' (borrowing stored energy to be replaced by aerobic means to be delivered later). There is, of course, no sudden sharp division between the energy sources utilized by contracting muscles; the percentages found in some research studies are shown in Table 10.3. What has just been described goes some way to explain a number of the features of muscle contraction noted in Table 10.1

Table 10.3 Relative contributions of aerobic and anaerobic processes to total energy during maximal muscular exercise of different durations

Duration of maximal exercise	Main energy source used	Anaerobic processes (%)	Aerobic processes (%)
10 seconds	ATP + creatine phosphate	83	17
1 minute	Glycolysis	60	40
2 minutes	Glycolysis and oxygen	40	60
5 minutes	Glycolysis and oxygen	20	80
10 minutes	Oxygen	9	91
30 minutes	Oxygen	3	97
1 hour	Oxygen	1	99

Modified from Berger, 1982.

A significant limitation for very prolonged muscle activity is the availability of the compounds from which energy is derived. In normally fed individuals, there are ample stores (sometimes rather over-ample in well fed populations!). In moderate exercise, much of the energy is drawn from carbohydrates, forming glucose used in the way described. In more prolonged exercise – such as long distance running – as the liver glycogen stores as well as muscle glycogen are used up, so more fatty acids are utilized in the TCA cycle. The stores of glycogen are never fully depleted because it is essential that the blood glucose should be kept at normal levels, since the nervous system and erythrocytes are entirely dependent on glucose for their energy needs. Thus, in starvation or prolonged exercise, the pattern of fuel usage changes to utilize the very large store of fatty acids in adipose tissue and, ultimately, in more severe starvation, proteins (i.e. body structure). The energy stored in fat is very much greater than all other energy storage; an example of the storage in kilojoules is given in Table 10.4.

Table 10.4 Energy reserves in adult males

Reserve	Energy (kJ)
Fat in adipose tissue	400 000
Protein in muscle	100 000
Glycogen in liver	800
Glycogen in muscles	1600
Glucose in blood	160

EFFICIENCY

The fact that contraction of muscle leads to the production of heat as well as mechanical energy has already been noted. Although the exact proportions vary in different situations, it is generally found that only some 25% of the available energy is converted to mechanical work; the remainder appears as heat. This is often described as being 'waste' heat and the mechanical work as being 'only' 25% efficient. Yet, in homeothermic organisms, such as humans, providing sufficient heat energy to allow chemical actions, notably enzymic reactions, to occur at or near their optimum temperature, is essential for life. Muscle metabolism provides a very significant part of the 200–300 W generated during the normal daily activity of a 70 kg man and may rise to 1000 W in strenuous activity. This means that there is a great deal of unwanted heat to be dissipated during vigorous exercise, which does lead to inefficiency since this heat energy is wastefully lost and often also leads to water loss in the evaporation of sweat. It may be noted that in cold circumstances, in which body heat is needed, it can be partly provided by muscle contractions that have no mechanical purpose, i.e. shivering.

The efficiency of a particular activity could be expressed as the energy consumption per unit time – i.e. the power in watts – compared with that found under different circumstances (e.g. what is the optimum, most efficient rate of walking?). It might be thought that this would be a fairly simple matter, since it is easy to measure the power of, say, an electric

Basic Biomechanics Explained

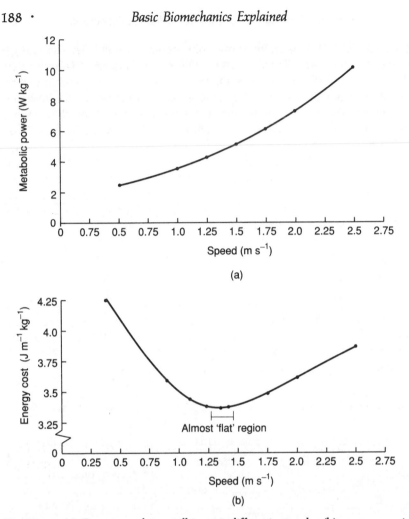

Fig. 10.2 (a) Power used in walking at different speeds; (b) energy cost of walking at different speeds.

motor. However, in humans, it is only possible to measure energy indirectly by measuring oxygen consumption. Further, it is difficult to separate the energy used for the actual muscle activity of walking from that used in basal metabolism, i.e. simply maintaining the body systems – digestion, respiration, circulation etc. – while the body is at rest. Of course, the activity of walking adds still further energy expenditure in that the circulatory and respiratory systems need to work harder, using more energy themselves.

If the energy consumption in watts per kilogram (including basal energy) is plotted against velocity, it is found, not surprisingly, that energy usage rises with the speed of walking. This is shown in Figure 10.2a, which is an approximation. Clearly, individuals of greater mass will use more energy. It can be calculated that a 70 kg man walking at $1.4\,\mathrm{m\,s^{-1}}$

would use 330 W. It is much more enlightening to consider the energy consumption per unit distance walked. When this is done, it is found that both very fast and very slow walking use more energy per metre than walking at moderate speeds. This is illustrated in Figure 10.2b, in which the energy usage cost in joules per metre per kilogram is plotted against speed. This result conforms with common experience and it is found that most adults required to walk fairly long distances (in which energy conservation is an important factor) automatically choose speeds around $1.3\,\mathrm{m\,s^{-1}}$ or $1.4\,\mathrm{m\,s^{-1}}$. Graphs like that shown in Figure 10.2b have been constructed from experimental results. The form of these graphs gives an equation relating the energy to the velocity with appropriate constants. An equation in SI units shows:

$$E = \frac{2.23}{\text{velocity}} + (1.26 \times \text{velocity})$$

where E is the energy consumption in joules per metre per kg of body mass and velocity is in metres per second (Whittle, 1991). From this equation all points on a graph like 10.2b can be derived and the values for individuals calculated from their weight.

Thus, a 70 kg man walking at $1.4\,\mathrm{m\,s^{-1}}$ would use:

$$\frac{2.23}{1.4} + 1.26 \times 1.4 \times 70 = 234.978 \text{ joules per metre}$$

and a 50 kg woman would use 167,842 joules per metre (or kilojoules per kilometre) walking at the same speed. Table 10.5 gives further figures; it can be seen that there is very little difference at speeds between $1.2\,\mathrm{m\,s^{-1}}$ and $1.45\,\mathrm{m\,s^{-1}}$. This is also represented in the flat part of Figure 10.2b. It should be stressed that the equation quoted above and Table 10.5 give mean values, but there is a very considerable range of individual variation. Additionally, variations are due to the circumstances in which the walk occurs, particularly the nature of the surface walked on. It can be seen that 1.33 metres per second (or 78 m per minute, or 4.68 km per hour or 2.908 miles per hour) is the most economical walking speed but, as indicated in Figure 10.2b and Table 10.5, speeds between about $1.2\,\mathrm{m\,s^{-1}}$ and $1.45\,\mathrm{m\,s^{-1}}$ (72–87 metres per minute) make very little difference and are nearly as economical.

Walking is an exceptionally economical means of locomotion, as noted above. At about $2.3\,\mathrm{m\,s^{-1}}$ in adults, walking changes to running because at that speed it is a more satisfactory gait, yet it is using about $5\,\mathrm{J\,m^{-1}\,kg^{-1}}$ compared with the $3.5\,\mathrm{J\,m^{-1}\,kg^{-1}}$ at $1.33\,\mathrm{m\,s^{-1}}$. Of course, as faster running occurs higher power is needed but the energy cost per metre remains almost the same. As explained above, the speed is limited by the power output of the muscles. Some of the discussion in Chapter 9 on the mechanisms of walking may now seem highly relevant. Walking is a very specific activity, which allows particularly economical locomotion. Thus,

Basic Biomechanics Explained

anything that interferes with the complex energy exchanges and predominantly isometric muscle activity of walking causes a faulty pathological gait and a considerable loss of function.

Table 10.5 Energy expended at different walking speeds and with different body weights

Velocity (m s^{-1})	Energy expended (J m^{-1})	
	70 kg	50 kg
1.1	238.928	170.35
1.26	235.020	167.872
1.33	234.674	167.624
1.4	234.98	167.842
1.55	237.419	169.585

A good deal of investigation has been carried out into abnormal or pathological gaits for obvious humanitarian and economic reasons. The general and expected findings are that any interference with joint mobility or muscle control leads to a slower and less economical gait. A single joint arthrodesis leads to measurable losses in energy efficiency. With more severe disabilities, such as amputation or hemiplegia, these are more evident and the slowing of the preferred walking speed makes the patient markedly less functional. For an account of some research findings on these matters, (see Waters and Yakura, 1990).

EXERCISE TESTING FOR CLINICAL PURPOSES

Much of the data described above have been elucidated from measurements of oxygen usage, carbon dioxide production, blood glucose levels and so forth, taken during exercise, but these are complex, expensive and often difficult to make. Various much simpler measurements, usually of the heart rate, have been used to provide some immediate assessment of the physiological response to aerobic exercise. The general principle involved in these tests is that a given amount of exercise will induce a greater physiological response, with a higher heart rate and a slower return to normal in the less physically fit. An example is the well known Harvard step test. In this, the subjects step on and off a step 51 cm (20 in) high at a rate of 30 steps per minute for five minutes and a pulse count is taken for 30 seconds starting one minute after exercise has ceased. If this pulse count for the full five minutes' exercise is above 100 beats per minute, the response is considered poor; if between 70 and 100 it is average, and below 70 good (Berger, 1982). An appropriate table of arbitrary scores can be used to compare the performance of those unable to complete the whole five minutes. This is quite a difficult test because of the height of the step and the fixed rate of work, so that it has been used largely for the assessment of relatively fit young males. More clinically applicable is the modified Tuttle–Dickinson pulse ratio test, which consists of stepping up and down on a 33 cm (13 in) step, 30 times per minute. The resting pulse, taken after sitting for one minute prior to the exercise, is divided into the total pulse count taken over two minutes immediately after the exercise. The result is called the pulse ratio. Since less fit individuals will have a higher post exercise heart rate, which will also take longer to return to normal, their pulse ratios will be higher; the normal value is considered to be 2.5. For many patients, this rate of exercise may be excessive and rates of stepping of 24 or 20 times per minute may be used with an extension of the time of stepping to two minutes (Karpovich, 1959). While such changes alter the outcome of the test, it is a valid index of variations in the aerobic capacity of the same patient undergoing the same test.

Table 10.6 Effort tolerance grading

1. Unable to hurry up hill	Mild disability
2. Unable to hurry on the level	
3. Unable to maintain a normal walking pace on level	Moderate disability
4. Unable to walk for 15 minutes ($\approx$400 m) without stopping	
5. Unable to walk 2/3 minutes ($\approx$100 m) without stopping	Severe disability

One of the main deficiencies of these tests is that the heart rate is likely to vary greatly for reasons unconnected with exercise (emotional stress, for example); also, repeated stepping up and down is an unusual activity for patients. A very useful assessment for walking, developed by James MacGregor (MacGregor, 1981) obviates these difficulties by using a measure called the Physiological Cost Index (PCI). In this, the difference between the resting heart rate and the heart rate monitored during walking is divided by the preferred walking speed. This gives the number of additional heart beats per metre while walking. For normal subjects, this averages 0.31 beats per metre and ranges (99% confidence limits) between 0.11 and 0.51 beats per metre. It is quite a sensitive measure of mobility impairment in a wide variety of circumstances and allows a distinction to be made between those whose walking efficiency falls within normal limits and those needing abnormally large metabolic efforts to maintain walking.

A plot of PCI against walking speed for a normal subject has a similar shape to Figure 10.2b in that the lowest PCI occurs at the preferred walking speed.

The walking ability of patients can also be graded roughly on a five-point scale, sometimes called an 'effort tolerance grading'. Normally, it is based on reported ability by the patient or carers. It is shown in Table 10.6.

OTHER ASPECTS OF PHYSICAL EXERCISE

The importance of an appropriate quantity and kind of bodily exercise is widely agreed. The damaging effects of insufficient physical movement are recognized in the atrophy of muscle and other tissues and overall loss of function. Equally, the beneficial effects of moderate exercise on the normal physiological processes are accepted. There is also agreement that these processes include not only the immune system but also brain function in that those undertaking moderate exercise tend to feel better and possibly function better at an intellectual level. (Although much quoted, it may be noted that the full quotation from Juvenal suggests that 'a healthy mind in a healthy body' should be prayed for, rather than it being cause and effect: 'orandum est ut sit mens sana in corpore sano'.) A recent study found that overall the population of England had surprisingly low levels of cardiovascular fitness – many middle-aged people were found to be unfit even for normal speed continuous walking on the level (The Health of the Nation, 1992). Even more alarmingly very low levels of aerobic fitness in school-age children have been noted.

Perhaps rather curiously, the benefit of exercise does not seem to correlate with the amount of exercise. It might be expected that the highly successful athlete would become 'superfit' in all ways, but this does not occur. There is good evidence that very vigorous training seems to depress the immune system in some way, allowing the athlete to suffer more often and more severely from infections. There is evidence that good marathon runners have lower than average lymphocyte counts and that there is a loss of T cells over the course of these races. While the reasons for this are unclear, alterations in hormone levels, psychological stress and decreases in the amino acid glutamine, which is needed for immune cell metabolism, have all been suggested (Sharp and Parry-Billings, 1992). Investigation of blood cell counts during and after prolonged (3 hours) physical activity has shown marked immediate changes. A small rapid increase in lymphocyte and platelet counts occurred at the start of exercise, rapidly subsiding at the end. A much greater but slower rise in granulocytes occurred subsiding even more slowly over 5–21 hours (Saradeth et al., 1991). These effects were more marked in the untrained. The degree of leucocytosis depended on the intensity and, to a lesser extent, the duration of the exercise.

It is hoped that this chapter has explained, to some degree, the fairly complex way in which human physical activity is maintained and some of the limiting factors. The term 'exercise' is used to cover everything from a single strong muscle contraction to prolonged low level activity, such as strolling in the street, and includes such vigorous actions as sprinting and marathon running. It has been shown that the physiological consequences of all these activities are often very different and that they are limited by different mechanisms. Further consideration is given to prolonged activity in part of Chapter 11.

11.   *Ergonomics*

Ergonomics – from 'ergon' (work) and 'nomos' (laws), the Greek derivation – is the study of human behaviour and interactions in relation to work and the working environment. It involves the design of appliances, technical systems and the workplace in such a way as to improve human performance, comfort, safety and health. While the term ergonomics is widely recognized, 'human factors engineering' is synonymously used in the USA and is, perhaps, more expressive. Like biomechanics, ergonomics involves contributions from many disparate fields, including anatomy, physiology, anthropometry, physics, engineering, industrial design and psychology. Biomechanics might well be regarded as a subdiscipline of ergonomics. As a summary of the meaning of ergonomics the title of a seminal book by E. Grandjean, *Fitting the Task to the Man* (1985), is apposite. This also emphasizes the idea of 'person centred' ergonomics. A particularly perceptive and well written overview of ergonomics and its relationship with physiotherapy (Foster, 1988) considers that physiotherapists are well placed to bring the benefits of human factor engineering to all levels of working organization, but need the authority provided by knowledge and understanding of the subject.

The areas covered by ergonomics can be classified broadly into studies involving:

1. *Human posture and positioning:* size and location of seats, height and reach in working positions, effects of prolonged standing or working overhead etc.
2. *Movement:* lifting and carrying, pulling and pushing, operating hand-held tools, energy costs of heavy work, muscular fatigue etc.
3. *Communication:* between people involving print size and layout, graphs and charts, symbols and readability, and between people and machines, such as visual displays or dials, visual display unit formats, warning lights etc.
4. *Design of the workplace and tools:* positioning of controls and displays, appropriate space, suitable size and efficient design of tools etc.
5. *Working environment:* appropriate levels of illumination, noise and vibration levels, temperature and humidity, air conditioning etc.

While the involvement of physiotherapists with the first two points is self-evident, there are many other situations in which impingement of ergonomics on therapy may occur. Rehabilitation is only completed on return to optimum functional activities, which include working. Understanding how physical limitations may affect working ability is essential. A number of aspects will be described in this chapter, which are considered to be of particular relevance to physiotherapy. Much ergonomic measurement is, of necessity, concerned with fitting the machine/instrument/seat etc. to the majority of the user population; 95% confidence limits are frequently employed. The disabled often fall outside these limits in some particular ability, such as arm reach mobility or muscle strength. Physiotherapeutic intervention might be directed specifically towards improving the ability needed for a particular work activity, such as sufficient grip strength to operate a tap. Alternatively, advice on adjusting the task may be appropriate, such as fitting a long lever to the tap to enable it to be turned on with less force. It must also be realized that many of the non-disabled find themselves outside design limits in some situations. (Tall men are as well aware of short beds and low doorways as short women are of high library shelves!) The sinistral population has to adapt to an almost entirely right-handed world. Designs are often only suited to a particular population. Many working controls have traditionally been based on male use only; for example, the pressure that can be exerted on a brake pedal has been found to be about 623 N for men but only half that force in women (Mortimer, 1974).

BODY SIZE: ANTHROPOMETRY

Body size and shape has already been addressed in Chapter 3. Some further details are given in Table 11.1 and also Figure 11.1, which elucidate some of the measurements. Attention is again drawn to the large variations between individuals; the mean measurements are given here. Furthermore, they are the mean measurements of a specific population — German adults in Table 11.1 — which are likely to differ slightly from other European or North American populations, and markedly from many other populations, for example, people from Thailand or Vietnam. The use of simple averages leads to the fallacious concept of an 'average person'. While there is a strong tendency, for example, for tall people to have long arms and vice versa, it is not possible accurately to deduce the size of one body part from another (Oborne, 1995). In spite of these provisos, the data presented here provide a useful base. (It may be noted that in Tables 11.1 and 11.2 and the discussion of reaches, the body height is that without shoes. Since shoes are normally worn in working situations, 2 cm, or more if high heels are in use, should be added.)

Some of the data in Table 11.1 can be compared with those obtained on men from other studies as shown in Table 11.2, to show that there is very little difference between the populations of the countries indicated. However, these data are now about 30 years old so that some increase in these averages will have occurred.

The mean differences between the sexes show up clearly in Table 11.1 in that the only measurement in women that is larger than that in men is the pelvic breadth. The shoulder breadth and hence arm span are very much greater in men.

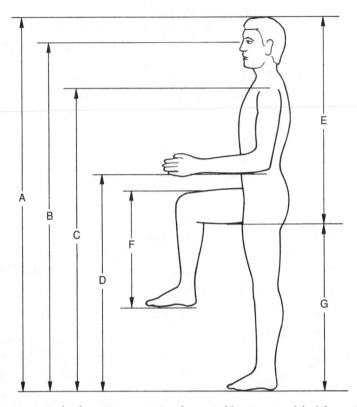

Fig. 11.1 Body dimensions; A–G refer to Table 11.1 (modified from Grandjean, 1985)

Table 11.1 Mean body dimensions of persons aged between 20 and 65 years (modified from Kroemer, 1964)

In Fig. 11.1	Body measurement	Men (cm)	Women (cm)
A	Standing height (unshod)	172	161
B	Eye level in standing	161	150
C	Shoulder height in standing	142	131
D	Elbow height in standing	106	97
E	Height in sitting	90	85
–	Span of arms	175	155
F	Sole of foot to knee	55	50
G	Sole of foot to popliteal space	45	43
–	Breadth of shoulders	45	41
–	Breadth of hips	35	37

These data were based on 15 700 men and 17 700 women from the Federal Republic of Germany.

Table 11.2 Mean values for males (cm)

	West Germany	USA	UK	France	Switzerland
Standing height	172	173	171	170	169
Sitting height	90	86	85	88	–
Elbow height in standing	106	106	107	105	104
Shoulder breadth	45	45	46	–	44
Breadth of hips	35	35	–	35	34

Data from various studies; modified from Grandjean, 1985.

What has been described is often called 'static' or 'structural' anthropometry in that it deals with the static circumstances of lengths, circumferences, body weight and so forth. This is distinct from 'functional' or 'dynamic' anthropometry, which deals with movement. This latter has been touched on in Chapter 6 in connection with the measurement of joint ranges of motion; reaches and working ranges would also be included.

The vertical reach is of great consequence in many situations; it obviously depends on the height and arm length of the subject. It further depends on what is meant by 'reach'. Thus, to place the hand flat on a shelf, the height of the shelf can be only about one seventh of the body height above the head (height × 1.14). For the fingertips to just touch the shelf it can be about 1/4 of the height above the head (height × 1.24). For something to be grasped, it can be at maximum about half way between the two foregoing measurements. Similarly, guidelines for arm reach in sagittal and horizontal planes suggest an average grasping distance of about 50 cm, but, of course, this varies with height and arm length.

POSTURE AND WORKING HEIGHTS

When work is done on a bench or table, the nature of the work dictates the body position, coupled with the height from the ground of the working surface. It is important to arrange the height of the worksurface to ensure a comfortable and appropriate posture for the worker. For precision work while standing, it is best to have the bench high enough to support the elbows, whereas, for light manual work, it should be lower to allow room for tools and materials. If heavy work is to be performed involving the weight of the upper body pressing on the tools, the bench should be lower still. Suggested heights (Grandjean, 1985) are shown in Table 11.3 and are based on elbow height in standing (see Table 11.1).

Table 11.3 Heights of bench for work in standing

Precision work, e.g. drawing	Light work with tools	Heavy work with weight applied
5–10 cm above elbow height	10–15 cm below elbow height	15–40 cm below elbow height

One of the major factors that determines the best height of the work surface is the distance from the eyes. Hence, for precision work the higher bench, noted in Table 11.3, brings the work closer to the eyes; between 10 cm and 30 cm is suggested (Dul and Weerdmeester, 1991/3). Since much close precision work is carried out at desks or tables, with the operator in a sitting position, the heights of the chair and the work surface are very important. Reading and writing require rather greater eye-to-work distances. The recommended table heights for seated work are: 90–110 cm for men doing precision work at close visual range and 10 cm less for women; 74–78 cm for men reading and writing and 4 cm less for women (Grandjean, 1985). For those using a keyboard, its thickness increases the effective height so that the table should be rather lower: 68 cm for men and 65 cm for women. All the foregoing suggested heights presuppose that the height of the operator's chair is fully adjustable. Sufficient space for the thighs beneath the desk is also important; adjusting the seat to be some 27–30 cm below the desk seems to be comfortable for the majority of users. In both sitting and standing, the head needs to be somewhat flexed at the neck to keep the work in the visual field. It has been found that the most comfortable head posture in sitting for the majority of workers was with the neck in some 17–29° of flexion. In standing, less flexion (8–22°) was appropriate (Grandjean, 1985). Keeping the neck posture correctly aligned has considerable implications for patients with cervical spondylosis and similar musculoskeletal disorders of the cervical region. Adjustments to desk, chair or work surface heights may be needed to ensure pain-free working.

POSTURE AND SEATING

Sitting has come to be regarded as a natural posture, due to the widespread use of seats and chairs, but it must be realized that it is a relatively recent development, postures such as squatting and crouching being more primitive. Seats have developed for different purposes, principally to provide support for resting in a more or less upright position and to provide a supported position for working. Compared with other upright postures sitting is less fatiguing and more metabolically economical. (It may be remarked, in passing, that seats have developed as status symbols, culminating in royal thrones. This status function persists in many modern circumstances; leather bound upholstery for company directors, better padded seats in first-class railway carriages or expensive seats in theatres.)

While sitting involves less isometric muscle work in the lower limbs than standing, it is necessary to stabilize the trunk so that there is still some muscle work for the legs and especially for the back muscles. The amount of work for these muscles depends on the posture of sitting; leaning back against a backrest, it is at a minimum but it becomes greater the more upright the posture (Andersson and Ortengren, 1974). It is believed that excessive periods spent in a poor sitting position may contribute to deterioration of the lower lumbar intervertebral discs, with consequent backache and perhaps associated sciatic pain. Certainly these discal pressures have been found to be higher in sitting than in standing, particularly so when the trunk is upright or bent forwards, whilst leaning back against a backrest is associated with lower intradiscal pressures (Andersson and Ortengren, 1974). The reason for these higher pressures would seem to be the change in lumbar spine posture from the standing position with a significant lordosis, to sitting, in which the lumbar vertebrae are vertically above one another or even in some flexion.

The purposes or reasons for sitting divide seats into three broad categories. First, easy chairs are for comfort and relaxation and are characterized by being well upholstered and having a backrest that allows the sitter to lean well back in a semi-reclining position. There is a maximum of support, which may include padded armrests and the seat is low enough to allow the legs to be outstretched somewhat, as the feet rest on the floor. These are for relaxation. Secondly, there are chairs suitable for work, the office or the laboratory. These need to provide stability while allowing free movement of the arms and, to some extent, the trunk. They allow further mobility by being free to rotate and by having castors. The third group are the multipurpose chairs that are a compromise and found in numerous places as chairs for sitting at a table or in waiting areas or lecture halls.

Chair dimensions must, of course, be appropriate to the populations that are to use them; the measurements suggested below apply to those described in Table 11.1.

Seat height: For an easy chair, 38–45 cm is suggested, whereas work and multipurpose chairs should be 43–50 cm (Oborne, 1995). As noted, the sitter in an easy chair is able to relax with the legs outstretched, while in the other chairs the feet are able to rest on the floor relieving uncomfortable pressure from the posterior surface of the thighs. It is widely recommended that working chairs should be made fully adjustable for height, particularly so that they may be adjusted for work surfaces as well as individual height.

Seat width: 40–43 cm is recommended for all types.

Seat depth: The distance from the front to the back of the seat of an easy chair is suggested as 43–45 cm, but 35–40 cm for a work chair. This should allow the seated person to use the backrest without the front edge of the seat pressing into the popliteal space.

Backrest height and width: The back support of easy chairs can be up to any height and may support the head. For work or multipurpose chairs, the height up from the seat varies and may be anything from 48 cm to 63 cm. There are good reasons for either shaping the backrest, so that the sacrum and the upper part of the gluteal region are accommodated, or omitting the lower 15 cm or so of the backrest to ensure that the lumbar and lower thoracic regions are supported. For many working chairs, the backrests are small and restricted to this area only to allow freedom of movement for the arms and shoulders. In all cases, the width should be about 35–48 cm.

Angle of the seat: This refers to the angle that the seat makes with the horizontal. Many easy chairs have a seat that is tilted backwards by 14–24°. This tilts the sitter on to the backrest, thus providing greater support, and, because it increases the area of contact, there is reduced local pressure. It also prevents the sitter from gradually slipping forward. This does not apply to the work chair, in which the sitter needs to lean forwards so that backward tilting would increase the spinal flexion needed and increase pressure of the front edge of the seat in the popliteal region. Work chairs, then, should have no tilt, or, as has been suggested (Mandel, 1976) they should slope forwards for up to about 15°. If forward tilted seats are used, it will be found that they need to be covered with material that gives a high coefficient of friction between the sitter and the seat to limit forward sliding.

Angle of the backrest: This, it is suggested, should be at an angle of around 108° to the seat (around 125° to the horizontal). The advantages of the tilted seat are enhanced by the tilted backrest providing added support and preventing forward sliding. For work chairs the angle should be rather more vertical.

Seat profiles, in 'sagittal' section, for an easy and a multipurpose chair are shown in Figure 11.2 to illustrate the general shapes found to be desirable. These were derived from the impressions of comfort from a number of subjects but, as can be seen, they conform to the recommended measurements.

Cushioning and upholstery: Padding helps to distribute the load, hence reducing pressure. This is especially important where high pressure is likely to occur under the ischial tuberosities. It also helps stability, up to a point, because the body is able to sink into it to some degree. However, if the cushioning is too soft, the body is unstable and extra muscle work is needed to maintain and adjust the position. As might be expected, softer cushioning is appropriate in an easy chair where a larger area of support is available than on work or multipurpose chairs. Some tests on seats have shown 'firmer' seats to be preferred.

Special seating: In order to prevent flexion in the lumbar spine while

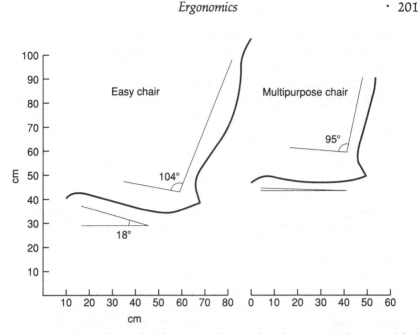

Fig. 11.2 Profiles of comfortable easy chair and multipurpose chair (modified from Grandjean, 1985).

seated, a Balans chair can be used. This has a forward sloping seat – of about 20° – and a knee support to prevent forward sliding. It cannot be used for long periods, due to pressure on the knees and the need to keep the legs in the same position. Subjects with and without low back pain were compared when using this seat over a one-hour period (Jackson, 1995). While little objective difference was found, the majority of subjects commented that the chair was quite comfortable. A pedestal stool consists of a high seat (65–85 cm) tilted forwards by 15–30°. This can be used to provide some support in a near-standing posture and is not unlike a shooting stick in function. For some working situations in which people change often from sitting to standing or for those with particular difficulty in rising from a normal chair, high stools have an advantage. The difficulty in rising from an easy chair often troubles the elderly and disabled. Besides the addition of arm rests at a suitable height, there are special chairs with seats that elevate and tip forward as the sitter rises. These chairs may be spring-operated and need to be adjusted for the weight of a particular patient, or they may be electrically operated and therefore needing connection to the mains. A hydraulically moved chair has also been described (Smith *et al.*, 1984) in which the seat raising is brought about by pumping a lever at the side of the chair.

A most important point to recognize in connection with prolonged sitting is the need for periodic changes of position. The proclivity for pressure sores to develop in those with loss of sensation or an inability to move is strong evidence. Comfortable seating often becomes uncomfortable after prolonged sitting if it restricts movement too much. The beneficial effects of regular and frequent changes of posture, including moving from sitting to standing, are becoming more widely recognized and will be further recommended.

MUSCULAR WORK

Static muscle work

From what has been described in Chapters 4 and 10 it is evident that prolonged muscle working requires an adequate blood flow. This is needed to supply the necessary oxygen and carbon compounds for muscle metabolism to proceed, as well as to remove the carbon dioxide and lactate. The rate of flow will need to be higher the harder the muscle is required to work. As an example, some muscle at rest has been found to have a rate of flow of 4 ml per minute per 100 g of muscle, whereas moderate work increases this to about 80 ml per min and heavy work to 150 ml per min per 100 g of muscle (Scherrer, quoted in Grandjean, 1985). When a muscle is contracting, the intramuscular pressure is increased, causing vessels in the muscle to be compressed, thus restricting the blood flow through them. This applies to all intramuscular vessels but most markedly to the soft-walled low pressure veins, venules and lymphatic vessels. When the muscle subsequently relaxes, the pressure is reduced, allowing the blood and lymph flow to be resumed. Since these vessels are valved, alternate compression and relaxation will effectively pump the contained fluid towards the heart. The pressure squeezes the fluid away only in the direction allowed by the valves and relaxation allows the filling of the vessel in the same direction. Thus, if a muscle is working rhythmically with the contractions lasting at most only a few seconds, the blood flow is enhanced and allows the muscle to continue in this way for long periods. If, on the other hand, the muscle contracts isometrically and continuously, the blood flow is inhibited so that the contraction cannot be maintained for long periods. The time for which a continuous isometric contraction can be held is inversely related to the force of the contraction. This is illustrated in Figure 5.11 and was also noted in Chapter 10. It follows that, if the muscle is to work statically for very long periods, it can only do so when generating forces of about 15–20% of its maximum. It is believed that at these low muscle tensions the blood flow is normal. It seems from Figure 5.11 that, when the muscle is working at 50% of its maximum, it can sustain the contraction for only a minute or so and the maximum force of contraction can occur for only about six seconds

All kinds of work involve some muscles in prolonged periods of isometric contraction. This includes those muscles needed to maintain an appropriate body posture. A familiar example is that of sawing wood. While it is possible to hold a small piece of wood firmly in one hand while sawing with the other, the static effort required by the holding hand and arm is so great that it is usual to fix the wood in some way. Simply holding it against a bench stop with the upper body weight applied through the holding hand is one way; holding it on a low trestle with the foot is another; or fixing it in a carpenter's vice or clamp, which frees the hand, is a third. For many working situations, some unusual posture needs to be maintained statically for long periods – bending over the work is often needed, for instance – which leads to fatigue in the stabilizing muscles. Many working situations are a mixture of static and dynamic work, such as lifting and carrying objects. These tasks are more efficiently and comfortably carried out if the static component can be kept to a low force. This can be achieved in various ways. To carry loads even short distances involves much static work, so trolleys or some other support are often used. Maintaining any posture involves some isometric muscle work, but this is normally minimized in several ways. As described earlier, the body segments can be balanced on one another so that very little muscle work is needed to hold the position. In many situations, the muscle is not working absolutely statically because of small to and fro movements, such as the sway in standing as described in Chapter 3. Many of the postural muscles are specialized for sustained low force contraction, having a large number of red type I slow twitch fibres as described in Chapter 4. Finally, different groups of muscle fibres are utilized at different times, allowing recovery from fatigue. Thus 'normal' postures can be maintained for very long periods with little fatigue but, if the posture involves greater muscle work – as occurs when working with the trunk bent or with the hips and knees semiflexed – then fatigue rapidly occurs and the posture cannot be continued for long. Similarly, working with the arms above the head, or held outstretched, is limited by the fatigue that occurs in the muscles of the shoulder girdle. While muscle fatigue has been discussed in Chapter 4, it is easily recognized in these situations as muscle pain. This may be temporary and relieved by a change of posture, but long term immobility in an unsuitable posture has been found to be associated with chronic aches and pains in those muscles that are doing excessive static work.

In summary, it is the static or isometric muscle activity in working situations that is often the limiting factor. Rhythmical muscular activity is much less stressful and hence can be continued for long periods without fatigue. This is widely recognized, if subconsciously, in the extensive use of methods of supporting and holding pieces of work and arranging working positions to suit the worker's comfortable posture. However, many working circumstances would benefit from consideration of the proportion of static muscle work and whether this can be reduced. It may be noted that improvements to working situations that have been investigated and found to be beneficial are, in essence, often ways of reducing the amount of static muscle work. The provision of backrests to working seats, as described above, is one example: the lower energy consumption found when school satchels were carried on the back compared with that found when carried in the hand, is another.

Dynamic muscle work

There has been much consideration of the forces that are appropriate for dynamic muscle work. Clearly, the absolute muscle force needed will depend on the working situation and there are many factors that will determine the muscle force available. Large forces will require the application of large, hence, strong, muscle groups; lifting heavy weights is done using the strong extensor muscles of the legs, as is described later. The way in which the muscles are used; concentrically or eccentrically, the degree of stretch, the rate of shortening, the state of training, the age and sex of the worker – all described in Chapter 4 – will help to determine the force available. Similarly, the direction of the applied force will decide whether the body weight can be made to contribute. In general, pulling and pushing are stronger in the vertical, and weaker when applied horizontally. Taking account of all these factors, the maximum available muscle force can be estimated but it is recommended that continuous working should be limited to 30% of this maximum, with short periods of up to 50%. However, in many situations, much higher forces, often nearer the maximum the worker can produce, are needed and are not inappropriate when coupled with proper rest periods.

The principles for the layout of working situations can be summarized:

1. Avoid static muscle work where possible;
2. Where static muscle loads must be endured they should be kept below 15% of maximum;
3. Avoid unsuitable postures by providing appropriate body support and positioning;
4. Dynamic work should be limited to within the muscular capability of the worker;
5. Avoid prolonged activity in one position.

HEAVY EXERTION AND ENERGY DEMANDS

Heavy work is intended to refer to physical work that is limited by the stress on the heart and lungs, and by nutritional requirements. The rate of work is limited by these factors, and therefore the total energy expended in a working day is also limited. While mechanization in developed countries has greatly reduced the numbers of people involved in such heavy manual work, it is still common in the building, forestry and haulage industries, as well as in agriculture.

The measurement of energy has been described in Chapter 1, from which it will be recalled that the joule is the preferred unit. The most usual method of energy measurement in humans is by the use of oxygen consumption, which can be fairly conveniently measured (about 20 kJ of energy are released for every litre of oxygen consumed, but this figure varies depending on the proportions of glucose (21 kJ), fat (20 kJ) and protein (18 kJ) utilized.)

Even when there is no visible movement, a great deal of activity is occurring in the body – breathing, digestion, heart pumping and much chemical reaction – so that energy is being consumed all the time. This is called the basal metabolic rate; it varies with age, sex, body weight and other characteristics, and correlates approximately with the surface area of the body. For a 70 kg man, it is usually within the range 5000–9000 kJ per day (Burton, 1994) with 7000 kJ being a reasonable average, which is about 81 kJ per second (i.e. 81 W). (It is instructive to realize that a person lying in bed could be converting energy at a very similar rate to that of the 75 W bulb in their bedside light!) Any activity, such as standing up, walking about, eating and drinking, raises this basal rate considerably and working activities involving vigorous muscular action raise it still further. This latter value of the energy involved in working activities (work energy) has been investigated and is naturally greater in more vigorous occupations. Table 11.4 shows some examples with approximate values for men and women; 'normal activities' refers to the energy used beyond the basal, but not connected to work.

Table 11.4 Approximate energy demands of various occupations (kJ per day)

Occupation	Men	Women
Very heavy work: lumber worker, narrow-seam coal miner	20 000	–
Heavy work: building worker, ballet dancer, agriculture worker	16 000	13 500
Moderate manual work: fitter mechanic, HGV driver, postal delivery	13 000	11 000
Light work: typist, bookkeeper, hairdresser	11 100	9 000
Normal activities	2 500	2 200
Basal metabolic rate (men 70 kg; women 60 kg)	7 000	5 850

Figures are approximate and modified from data from Grandjean, 1985.

It can be seen from Table 11.4 that the heaviest work involves an increase of about 10 000 kJ over the basal-plus-normal activity rate and this – perhaps up to 22 000 kJ – seems to be the maximum that can be sustained as a regular daily activity. Much larger exertions can be made over a day or so. Energy consumptions of up to 40 000 kJ or more may occur in sport or strenuous mountaineering and in military training. There are many compromise situations in which heavy work exceeding 20 000 kJ is maintained over a few days, or even a few weeks, with succeeding slack periods. This is the situation in many seasonal occupations, especially agriculture.

These figures represent the total energy per day – i.e. over 24 hours – but this is made up of periods of much greater energy output interspersed with periods during which the energy usage is at, or close to, the basal metabolic rate, for example, during sleep. Further, almost all occupations or activities are not carried on continuously but involve frequent periods of relative rest. The energy cost of various activities has also been researched. The energy cost of walking was considered in Chapter 10 and the 70 kg man walking at 1.4 m s^{-1} was found to consume some 330 W. About two thirds of this would be accounted for by the act of walking being beyond the basal and normal rates. Such a subject walking for four hours would cover about 20 km (12.5 miles) using some 1188 kJ per hour (330 W = 0.33 kJ per second; 0.33 × 3600 = 1188); thus a total of 4752 kJ would be used in the four hours, of which about 1600 kJ might be used without walking. The additional 3150 kJ might seem rather a small figure, since walking 20 km in a day is reasonably equivalent to a moderate working day, perhaps the part of a postman's round done on foot. It must be realized that this refers only to walking on flat, even ground and ignores the many other associated activities. (Real postmen will explain that much extra energy is utilized in walking up hills, handling parcels and, perhaps, avoiding territorial dogs!) It must also be understood that walking at this pace is a particularly economical activity. In passing, slimmers may be interested to note that the extra 3150 kJ used in walking 20 km could be supplied by 197 grams of glucose (glucose supplies approximately 16 kJ per gram) or 81 grams of fat (fat supplies approximately 39 kJ per gram). Walking uphill uses much more energy than walking on the flat but, naturally, depends on the slope and the walking speed. Some data on this and other activities are given in Table 11.5, but it must be recognized that these are examples rather than exact measurements and depend on how the activity is performed.

Table 11.5 Rate of energy consumption for various activities (about 110 W are due to normal and basal activity)

Activity	Rate of energy consumption (W)
Walking at 1.4 m s^{-1} (or 5 km h^{-1}) on level	330
Climbing 16% slope rising at 11.5 m min^{-1}	689
Cycling at 16 km h^{-1}	473
Hammering with 4.4 kg hammer: 15 vertical strikes per minute	620
Shovelling: throwing 2 m horizontally and 1 m vertically at 10 shovels per min	654
Sawing wood with two-handed saw at 60 double strokes per minute	738

Modified from Grandjean, 1985

The higher work rates shown in Table 11.5 are rarely maintained for long periods – the 654 W of shovelling would lead to the consumption of over 2350 kJ per hour if done continuously – so that it tends to be performed with rest periods and a much lower hourly energy consumption results.

While high levels of work are undesirable and even damaging (see note in Chapter 10 on the effects of vigorous athletic training on the immune system) so too are low levels. The sedentary life being provided in industrialized countries leads to much underutilization of body functions, with deleterious effects on many systems, the most obvious being the tendency to obesity and associated coronary and circulatory diseases. It is suggested that healthy occupations should involve a daily energy consumption of 12 500–14 500 kJ (approximately 3000–3500 kcal) for a man and about 10–15% less for a woman. Many occupations may not reach this level (see Table 11.4), but the total energy consumption can be increased by appropriately energetic leisure activities.

CLIMBING STAIRS

Climbing stairs is a universal activity, which can become difficult for the disabled or the infirm. The structure of suitable staircases has long been described by a formula in which the sum of the tread depth and twice the tread height is 60 cm (or 64 cm) (see Fig. 11.3). Staircases can be made with different slopes by using this formula and there is evidence that a slope of around 30° is the most efficient in that it leads to the least consumption of energy. Other angles of slope are not very different in efficiency terms but cause variations in the gait used for climbing. Clearly, body size, especially height, is an important determinant of the gait that can be used on a particular flight of stairs. A study of women climbing steep and shallow stairs (but within the specifications of a building code) found that faster stepping rates were associated with the steeper stairs (and, as expected, shorter subjects), but subjects moved faster on the shallower steps (Livingstone *et al.*, 1991). They also noted that subjects adjusted to differing stair dimensions principally by varying the amount of knee flexion. It has been shown (Corlett *et al.*, 1972) that the physiological cost in terms of heart rate and oxygen consumption is always less for stairs than for ramps of equivalent slope. Stairs, however, require a special gait, as noted in Chapter 9, and are unsuitable for children's pushchairs, wheelchairs and trolleys.

While the formula, noted above and shown in Figure 11.3, has been widely used it can lead to the provision of extremely long or extremely narrow tread depths. These latter are unsatisfactory because there is insufficient space for the shod feet of taller subjects. Investigations of user preference (Irvine *et al.*, 1990) found that the optimum was a riser height of 18.3 cm with a tread depth of approximately 28–30 cm, as shown in Figure 11.3.

For stability while climbing and descending stairs, two other points

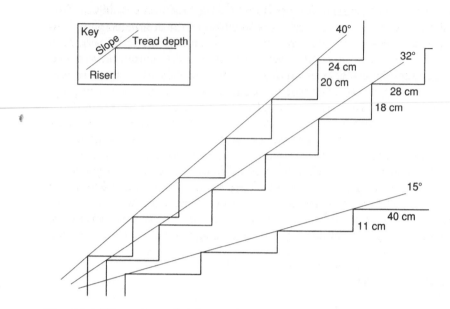

Fig. 11.3 Dimensions of stairs.

need to be considered. First, the coefficient of friction between the feet of the user and the tread surface and also between any carpeting or matting and the step surface. Slipping of the foot on the surface or the movement of loose matting on the step can cause accidents. Secondly, a handrail should be provided; this should be shaped to allow proper gripping and be a suitable height above the stairs (90 cm has been recommended).

LIFTING AND BACK PAIN

Lifting heavy weights is a suspected potent cause of back pain and disability. Much research has been conducted in working situations into the links between the type and amount of lifting and the incidence of back problems. There seems to be a strong relationship between the number of back injuries reported and the number considered by the sufferers to be due to lifting in a range of different occupations. While this does not mean that lifting caused the back injury, it suggests a link. Similarly, it has been found that back troubles occur more frequently and lead to longer periods of absence in heavy work than in light work. Heavy work refers to labouring, farming and other occupations in which heavy lifting may occur, such as nursing. However, the relationship is far from simple and much variation occurs with age, sex, the nature of the lifting performed and many other factors. Further, similar back complaints occur in those who do no lifting at work. One point of great importance is that less back pain seems to occur in those whose occupations involve much variation and not being restricted to long periods of sitting, standing or lifting. This point has been noted in connection with sitting, with prolonged periods in one posture being both uncomfortable and damaging. The human body is not well adapted to prolonged periods in any one position, or, it would seem, to repetitive identical activity (see later). Much lifting and carrying without other intervening activity would seem to be similarly damaging.

The pain in the back associated with excess lifting is usually considered to be due to a lesion of one of the lower lumbar intervertebral discs. Although the disc itself is insensitive (having no nerves), if it degenerates and allows a posterolateral herniation to press on adjacent spinal nerves, local and referred pain, paraesthesia and sometimes muscle weakness can result. Degeneration or other disorders of the disc may also allow excessive stress to be applied to adjacent ligaments and facet joint capsules, which are extensively innervated. It therefore seems appropriate to consider the structure and some mechanical features of the intervertebral disc at this point. This should be considered in conjunction with the discussion on spinal mechanics in Chapter 12.

The intervertebral disc

The intervertebral disc consists of a central fluid mass called the nucleus pulposus surrounded by a laminated fibrocartilaginous structure – the annulus fibrosus. The arrangement of fibres of the latter are shown in Figure 11.4a. The whole structure is sandwiched between hyaline cartilage plates, which connect it to adjacent vertebrae (Fig. 11.4b). The nucleus pulposus is a colloidal gel of water-absorbing glucosaminoglycan molecules and it has a water content of about 70% (Jensen, 1980). This makes it nearly incompressible, so that when the vertebrae are pressed together the nucleus bulges laterally, putting circumferential tension on the annulus fibrosus. This stretches the whole annulus, altering the orientation of the fibres, making them more oblique as well as stretching the fibres themselves and storing energy in the elastic distortion. The disc can thus act as a shock-absorber by converting compression forces on the spine to radial forces, which are resisted by the elasticity of the annulus fibrosus. The disc is prestressed in that, even with no outside compression force on the spine, the nucleus is under a pressure of some 10 newtons per square centimetre (Nachemson, 1960). This is considered to be due to the elastic properties of the ligamentum flavum (Nachemson and Evans, 1968). This concept of supporting compressive forces by circumferential tension will be found again in the mechanism of human lifting. The annulus fibrosus is connected to the anterior and posterior longitudinal ligaments at its periphery as well as to the edges of the vertebral bodies. More centrally, it is attached to the cartilaginous plates. Thus, it provides a strong but flexible union for adjacent vertebrae.

The arrangement also allows some limited motion between each pair of vertebrae. In flexion, the anterior part of the annulus is compressed, while

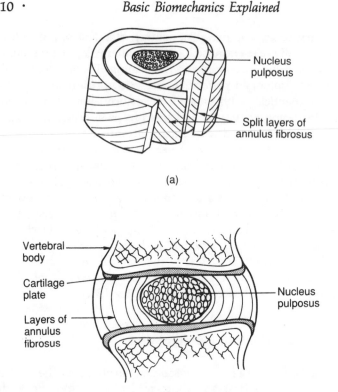

Fig. 11.4 Simplified representation of the intervertebral disc: (a) arrangement of fibres in the annulus fibrosus; (b) coronal section.

the posterior part is stretched, and vice versa in extension. The range of such movement is highly variable between individuals, but 15° might be typical for the lower lumbar region. Side flexion causes stretching and compression of the disc on opposite sides in the same manner but with only some 6° of movement at this level (Frankel and Nordin, 1980). Rotation stretches those annular fibres positioned at an angle, causing them to be elongated, although rotation in the lumbar region is negligible.

The changes in degeneration of the disc are considered to lead to a weakened, drier and less elastic structure. Partial rupture in the posterolateral part of the disc can lead to herniation and hence pressure on adjacent nerves. This may result from excessive compression forces applied to an already degenerate disc. It is also suggested that excessive prolonged loading of the discs may be a contributing cause of the degeneration. Study of the intradiscal pressure in different circumstances has been conducted and has led to advice regarding posture and lifting. That annular fibre ruptures occur is less surprising when it is noted that the tension force in the posterior part of a lumbar disc has been estimated to be four or five times that of the axial compression load (Nachemson, 1960). The intradiscal pressures in various postures and during various activities have been found for the third lumbar disc and are shown in Table 11.6. The pressures are expressed as a percentage of the pressure in standing. It can be seen that pressures in sitting are relatively high compared with standing or slow walking. The high pressures generated by lifting weights, especially with the back flexed, are also shown. It will be noted that the intradiscal pressures are quite low in standing and barely raised by slow walking. Unsupported sitting, however, leads to a marked increase. The reasons for this difference are considered to be, first, the higher tension in the abdominal muscles in standing, and thus the greater intra-abdominal pressure (explained below), and secondly, perhaps, the activity of the psoas major muscle, which stabilizes and thus compresses, the lumbar spine in sitting (Jensen, 1980). .

Table 11.6 Intradiscal pressure in third lumbar disc as a percentage of that found in standing

Position	Percentage pressure in standing
Standing	100
Supine lying	25
Side lying	75
Supine lying with legs supported (semi-Fowler position)	35
Side flexion of trunk 20°	133
Forward flexion of trunk 20°	150
Standing upright with 10 kg weight held in each hand	142
Unsupported sitting	140
Sitting bending forward 20°	185
Activities	
Walking slowly	107
Lifting 20 kg weight with knees bent and back straight	244
Lifting 20 kg weight with knees straight and back bent	380
Supine lying, bilateral straight leg raise	150
Prone lying hyperextension	180

Data from Grandjean, 1985 and Jenson, 1980; based on Nachemson, 1976.

When the whole spine is bent, say flexed, the anterior part is compressed while the posterior part is stretched. The discussion in Chapter 2 and also Figure 2.7 are pertinent to this point. Thus, during forward flexion, the anterior parts of the discs are compressed, while the posterior spinal ligaments are stretched. As these structures – the posterior longitudinal ligament, the ligamentum flavum and the interspinous and supraspinous ligaments – have greater stiffness than the disc, greater stress (force) occurs in them than in the disc (Radin *et al.*, 1992). As the discs deform more easily, the compression force is spread over a larger area and thus has a lower value. The axis in which neither compression nor stretch occurs is moved backwards (see Fig. 2.7). The ligaments are at different distances from the axis of movement; if they were mechanically identical, the more distant interspinous and supraspinous ligaments would be the most stretched and thus the most stressed. It is suggested that these structures have different elastic moduli so that, although the deformation of each ligament may differ during bending, the stresses are similar and the load is thus shared equally in all posterior ligaments (Radin *et al.*, 1992). The posterior spinal muscles perform a similar function during forward bending of the trunk by contracting eccentrically and sharing the stress with the posterior ligaments. Electromyographic studies have shown that usually the erector spinae muscles are slightly active during quiet standing, and active during flexion, but completely inactive in full flexion when the tension appears to be in the posterior ligaments only.

Straightening up from the fully flexed position leads to the reverse process. Curiously, even with some weight in the hands, the erector spinae do not always become active in the initial part of the movement of extension (Basmajian, 1974). This shows the reliance placed on the posterior spinal ligaments in flexion and ties in with the proclivity for injury when lifting in this posture.

Calculations of the compression forces exerted on the disc and vertebra during lifting, based on the weight of the upper body, the weight being lifted, the necessary force generated by the extensor muscles and their respective distances from the disc, suggest that the amount of weight lifted in moderately athletic weightlifting would be sufficient to cause vertebral fractures (Frankel and Nordin, 1980) (see also Chapter 12). Since this does not occur, there must be another mechanism to take a significant amount of the weight. This mechanism is the use of intra-abdominal pressure to help in the support. The abdominal cavity is effectively a fluid-filled chamber, so that pressure applied at any point will be transmitted equally in all directions. Thus, compression of the cavity by the simultaneous contraction of all the abdominal muscles, the diaphragm and the pelvic floor muscles, resists any force tending to approximate the rib cage (diaphragm) to the pelvis (pelvic diaphragm), as occurs in lumbar spine flexion. The mechanism, shown in Figure 11.5a, can be likened to a water-filled plastic bag or rubber balloon supporting a heavy book on a surface. If squeezed by hand on all sides, the bag will lift the book upwards or support a heavier one (Fig. 11.5b). As already noted, it is the same principle as that of the intervertebral disc providing support by a fluid nucleus pulposus being squeezed by an elastic annulus fibrosus. While the intra-abdominal pressure that occurs during lifting is not particularly high, two factors make it significant. First, the relatively large areas involved and, secondly, the considerable distance in front of the disc at which it is applied. This explains why the abdominal muscles contract and the breath

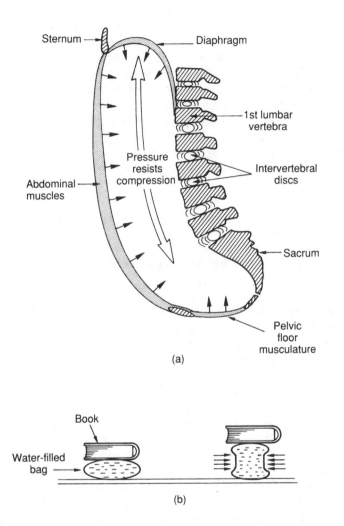

Fig 11.5 (a) Sagittal section of abdominal cavity; (b) squeezing a water-filled bag to support a weight.

is held during heavy lifting. It is thought that this mechanism becomes increasingly important with heavier loads and in dynamic lifting when the load has to be accelerated rapidly upwards (Frankel and Nordin, 1980). It also explains why inguinal or other hernias sometimes occur as a consequence of lifting; the increased pressure forces tissues through a weakened region of the abdominal wall. The traditional use of wide, tight belts as part of the equipment for occupations involving heavy lifting, such as heavy digging, and for competitive weight-lifting, is presumably an aid to raising the intra-abdominal pressure.

Heavy lifting

Heavy lifting refers to loads that are a significant proportion of the body weight; about a quarter of body weight is a reasonable suggestion. Lighter loads are often lifted by healthy subjects with little difficulty and with little risk of injury. Heavier loads can lead to considerable compression of the intervertebral discs, stretching of the ligaments and, perhaps, damage to the spinal facet joints. If loads are lifted with the back bent and the knees straight, the compression of the disc is very great, but if the knees are flexed and the lumbar spine kept nearly straight the intradiscal pressure is less, as noted above in Table 11.5. For heavy lifting, then, the 'leg lift' – as it is sometimes called – should be used. This is described as follows:

> The knees and hips are bent but the lumbar spine is maintained straight and nearly upright;
> The object to be lifted is held as close to the body as possible;
> The back extensors and abdominal muscles are contracted (the breath is held during the lift).

This, and the 'back lift', which is not advised, are illustrated in Figure 11.6. For the routine lifting of heavy objects, such as occurs in industrial situations, rules have been developed to take account of the variables. The method developed by the National Institute for Occupational Safety and Health (1981) of America can be used to decide what load is the maximum that should be lifted in unsuitable lifting conditions. It presumes a maximum load of 23 kg in optimal lifting conditions, which is reduced in less favourable conditions. The horizontal and vertical distances between the body and the load, the vertical distance the load is lifted, the lifting frequency in lifts per minute, and the way the load is grasped, are all taken into account and inserted into a formula to produce the maximum recommended weight limit. Due to the complexity of this analysis, appropriate computer software is available using the method. The analysis presupposes that the lifting posture can be freely chosen, which is often not the case.

Lifting heavier loads than 23 kg is common, and includes lifting and handling in both care and treatment situations. Two carers lifting an adult patient means that they are lifting around half their own body weight and often more. Further, it is often difficult to meet optimum lifting recommendations in such situations, particularly in positioning the feet of the lifter. Advice on lifting given to therapists and nurses is sometimes reduced to simplified rules without explanation of the mechanisms involved. This practice is often unhelpful.

In executing a 'leg lift' of either a heavy object or a patient, the compression force on the spine is lessened the nearer the load is to the trunk, since the torque exerted by the load is thus reduced. This has a very significant effect. The way in which the load is grasped is important. For

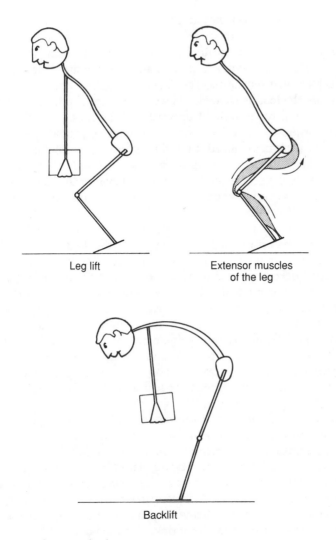

Leg lift

Extensor muscles
of the leg

Backlift

Fig. 11.6 Lifting methods.

many objects, the provision of suitably sized and sited (40–50 cm off the
floor) handles is helpful. For large, often irregularly shaped objects like the
human body the area of contact should be as large as is feasible. This
reduces the local pressure for both the lifter and the patient. Thus, the
whole hand and the forearm may be used. For some patient lifts, the area
of contact is further increased by the patient's arm pressing on the lifter
(i.e. the 'shoulder lift'). The position of the lifter's back is 'set', with the
lumbar spine near-straight; this posture is held during the lift so that the
erector spinae and abdominal muscles are contracting isometrically. These
muscles are contracted prior to the lifting action to ensure that ligaments
are protected. The greater force capability of isometric over concentric

contraction has already been noted. Naturally, during the lift, the pelvic floor muscles and the diaphragm will also be isometrically contracted to maintain a relatively high intra-abdominal pressure. Numerous other muscles may also be involved, particularly to stabilize the ribs and scapulae, such as latissimus dorsi. The arm and shoulder girdle muscles are also 'set' before the load is moved. Thus the load, trunk and arms become effectively one unit to be moved upwards by the legs. This allows the strong extensor muscle groups of the lower limbs to provide the vertical movement. It must be realized that during normal activities, such as stepping up a kerb, the whole body weight can be lifted by the extension of one leg (see discussion on climbing stairs in Chapter 9). Thus, the lift is effected by the powerful knee and hip extensor muscles, which are customarily used for raising the body weight vertically in stepping and jumping. It will be recognized that these principles are embodied in the techniques for competitive weightlifting, with the legs being used to accelerate the weights upwards in two stages and then momentarily held with all joints 'locked' in an extended position. The use of a belt and breath-holding is also evident. The large weights lifted are close to the theoretical limits and hence unsafe without training in the correct technique. A lift conducted in this way rightly avoids any foot movements, and rotatory or side movements of the trunk. This ensures that the weight is distributed more or less evenly between the two feet and throughout the trunk. Rotary motion during lifting is considered a potent cause of back injury, probably because it allows high forces to be localized in one region.

It should be understood that lifting different kinds of objects will need somewhat different techniques. What has been said above is intended to illuminate the principles. For example, objects being lifted from the floor may be so bulky as to prevent them being placed between the lifter's bent knees, thus forcing the lifter further from the object and greatly increasing the force on the spine. Large, solid objects may be tipped on one edge or a corner to allow lifting. For long, heavy objects like metal pipes or concrete posts, lifting one end first (thus lifting only half the weight initially, which lessens as the pipe is moved upright; see Chapter 5) allows the lifter to support the object at its centre of gravity; this part has now been raised, easing the lift. It may even have been raised sufficiently to need no further lifting if the pipe is long enough. Lifting patients is a special problem because the primary concern must be for the comfort and security of the patient. Several different techniques, using two lifters, are recommended for lifting and moving patients (see Health and Safety Executive, 1992b).

As stated in the introduction to this chapter, the areas of study covered in ergonomics include much of importance in the study of communication between people and between people and machines, as well as consideration of the working environment. There is much more to the application of ergonomics than attention to posture, sitting and lifting, although these are important (Foster, 1988). In advocating further education in ergonomics for therapists, Foster goes on to say, 'The aim [should be] ... to equip the therapist with an overall awareness of the occupational scene in which their own expertise of rehabilitation and education of movement can be applied.' This chapter has done no more than provide a taste of this important area of study.

12.   *Some biomechanical explanations*

EXPLANATIONS AND EXAMPLES

This final chapter contains a number of separate, distinct and unrelated items, which illustrate and draw upon the principles discussed in the previous chapters. Some of these are extremely simple and it is hoped that the reader will not feel that their intelligence is being insulted, but recognize that elementary applications are often a necessary step towards a fuller understanding.

THE SHAPE AND MOTION OF SYNOVIAL JOINTS

In synovial joints, one articular surface moves with respect to another and they are often considered superficially to act as a simple mechanical joint. The naming of joints, in classifying them as 'hinge' or 'ball and socket' for example, encourages this view. In reality, synovial joint surfaces are never perfectly flat or sections of a perfect sphere or cylinder, but are always parts of ovoid surfaces. Often, they are multiple ovoids and may be either convex or concave, or in some joints both, when they are sellar (saddle shaped). A convex ovoid surface is readily visualized by thinking of part of an eggshell, larger eggs having a less sharp curvature and vice versa. Similarly, the inside of the shell is a concave ovoid surface.

The two surfaces of joints do not fit exactly with one another except (usually) at one extreme of motion, called the 'close-packed' position. For all other positions – 'loose packed' positions – the articular cartilages of both surfaces are in contact over only part of their surface area. The gap between them is, of course, filled with synovial fluid. This arrangement is thought to be important for joint lubrication (see Chapter 6), and perhaps cartilaginous nutrition. The most loose-packed position of many joints is near the middle of their functional range, which is a position in which the extra-articular tissues are often sufficiently lax to allow separation of the joint surfaces by gentle traction if the muscles are relaxed. In close packing, on the other hand, the surfaces are firmly applied to one another and fit together, with the ligaments in tension. The conjunct rotation that occurs tends to 'spiralize' the ligaments and capsule, effectively 'locking' the joint. Many joints operate functionally very near, but not at, their fully close-packed position when stability is needed. This allows the elasticity of tissues to resist further movement in one particular direction, providing stability and saving muscle effort, e.g. the extended knee joint in standing. Table 12.1 lists the close-packed and most loose-packed positions of a number of joints.

Table 12.1 Close- and loose-packed positions of some joints

Joint	Close-packed position	Most loose-packed position
Hip	Extension and medial rotation	Semiflexion
Shoulder	Abduction and lateral rotation	Mid-abduction, mid-flexion
Knee	Extension	Semiflexion
Wrist	Dorsiflexion	Semiflexion
Ankle	Dorsiflexion	Mid-plantarflexion

When a convex joint surface moves on a concave one, or vice versa, and is not in contact over all its area, it can move in three ways. It may:

Slide — a translational motion;
Roll — like a wheel on a road;
Spin — rotate around an axis perpendicular to the surface.

These are all illustrated in Figure 12.1. In normal joint motion, these movements usually occur in combination. It can be seen at once that a combination allows greater joint angulation without an increase in the area of the surfaces involved. The knee joint provides an easily visualized example. During extension, the femoral condyles roll forwards on the tibial surface, but slide backwards at the same time. Towards the end of the movement the medial femoral condyle moves backwards even further, imparting a degree of medial rotation or spin around a vertical axis (see 'The knee' below).

THE SPINAL COLUMN

The biomechanics of the spinal column is inevitably highly complex, due to the irregular shape and multiplicity of the different muscular and gravitational forces that act upon it. Despite this, some useful insights can be gained by considering various simple mechanical aspects of the spinal column.

If the spine is considered as a flexible column designed to support axial compression loads, several features are at once evident. First, the size of the vertebrae of which it is composed generally enlarge towards the lower weightbearing segments. This is very reasonable, since the lower part must bear the most weight and be subjected to the highest stresses. Secondly, considered in a coronal plane, the column is, more or less,

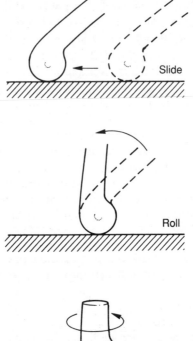

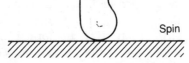

Fig. 12.1 Three types of motion in synovial joints.

straight. Common experience of long slender flexible columns indicates that they will support quite large forces until, at a critical force, they quite suddenly buckle. This can be readily recognized in a tube of rolled-up paper. This form of structural failure is known as 'Euler buckling' (pronounced 'oiler') because it was first analysed by Leonhard Euler (1707–1803), who developed a formula to describe the load at which the long strut will buckle. In general, this load is proportional to the elasticity and cross-sectional area of the column and inversely proportional to the square of it's length. Strictly, the load at which the column will buckle equals:

$$\pi^2 \; \frac{E \times I}{L^2}$$

in which E = Young's modulus of elasticity, I = the moment of inertia of the cross-section and L = the length of the column (Gordon, 1978). This is the simplest situation in which both ends of the column are free to move in one plane, but, if rotation of one end is prevented, the critical buckling force is greater. If both ends are fixed, it is greater still. It has been found that the critical force for buckling of the isolated vertebral column (from a cadaver devoid of musculature) is very low indeed, at about 20 N. With the ribs, sacrum and muscles attached, it has been calculated to be around 350 N (Radin *et al.*, 1992), which is about equivalent to the weight of the upper body. Clearly, in the living body, spinal stability is dependent on the contractions of the trunk musculature. As far as lateral stability is concerned, the vertebral column has often been likened to a ship's mast stabilized by taut rigging in the form of muscles. As the lower end of the vertebral column is fixed via the sacrum and the pelvis, the critical load to cause buckling is increased over that predicted by the simple Euler equation. The vertebral column is not a straight rod in the sagittal plane but bent into a thoracic kyphosis and lumbar and cervical lordoses in standing adults. It is impossible to have spinal bending in a plane at right angles to these curves without some additional rotation about a longitudinal spinal axis. This is not a special anatomical property of the spine, but will be found to occur in any long flexible rod; bending in two planes perpendicular to one another leads to rotation. Thus, lateral deviation (scoliosis) is inevitably associated with rotation between vertebrae. In pathological scoliosis, the greatest rotatory deformities are in the thoracic region, which allows much more rotation than the lumbar region. When the bent spine is being considered, the load is no longer axial but is now acting to increase the bend. This applies both when the spine is flexed, as in lifting from the floor, and when markedly side-flexed, as in severe pathological scoliosis. In these situations, part of the spine effectively becomes a cantilever, that is a beam, one end being fixed and the other supporting the load. Beams in this situation bend until the stress in the beam balances the applied load, the upper region of the beam being stretched and the lower compressed.

Thus, supporting the body weight through the vertebral column is largely a matter of maintaining the column of bones in an orientation that supports the axial loads and resists buckling. This appears to be achieved by complex muscle arrangements that allow the adjustment of tension and position between individual vertebrae. The adjacent vertebral arches are united by numerous muscle slips: intertransversarii, between the transverse processes; interspinales, between the spines; rotatores, between transverse processes and laminae, the semispinalis and the deeper fasciculi of the multifidus passing from mamillary or transverse processes to the spines of the vertebrae above. Further, many muscle fasciculi bridge over one, two or three vertebrae, the more superficial multifidus and semispinalis, for example. The variety of angles at which force can be exerted on the vertebrae by these muscle arrangements, coupled with the evidence that these muscles (or at least some of them) have a significantly larger number of muscle spindles than the major superficial back muscles, supports their role in control (Norris, 1995).

During standing, the centre of gravity of the upper part of the body usually falls anterior to the transverse axis of motion of all spinal

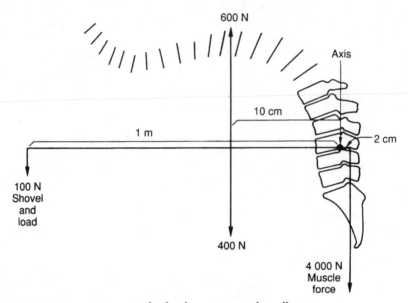

600 N

Axis

10 cm

1 m

2 cm

100 N
Shovel
and
load

400 N

4 000 N
Muscle
force

Fig. 12.2 Forces acting on the lumbar spine in shovelling.

segments, thus tending to produce flexion. This is counterbalanced by the elasticity of the posterior ligamentous structures and passive elastic components of the posterior muscles. The intervertebral discs also contribute, as described in Chapter 11. Sway occurs in standing, as noted in Chapter 3, which is associated with intermittent activity in the erector spinae, abdominal and psoas muscles, as well as (it is thought) with activity in the deep intersegmental muscles for the reasons given above. The activity in different muscle groups varies between individuals and may be associated with the particular standing posture adopted.

LIFTING AND THE LUMBAR SPINE

It is intended that this section should be considered in conjunction with the discussion on lifting in Chapter 11. Various analyses of lifting have been made by considering the spine as a cantilever fixed at the hips and loaded through the arms. The forces on the lumbar spine can be estimated; the example illustrated in Figure 12.2 is based on McNeil (1981). The subject is considered to be shovelling. The mass of the shovel and contents are estimated to be 10 kg centred 1 m from the axis of motion of the lumbar spine. Half the body weight of 80 kg is considered to act 10 cm from the lumbar centre of motion. These flexing forces are balanced by the extensor musculature acting 2 cm behind the axis and the intra-abdominal pressure of an estimated 600 N at 10 cm in front of the axis. Thus, taking the acceleration due to gravity as 10 m s^{-2} for convenience, the force of the shovel and contents equals 100 N and that of the upper body weight of 40 kg equals 400 N. Taking moments about the lumbar spine centre:

$$\Sigma -(100 \times 1)-(400 \times 0.1) + (600 \times 0.1) + (\text{muscle force} \times 0.02) = 0$$

thus muscle force $= 4000$ N
To find the compression force in the tissues and lumbar spine 'R':

$$\Sigma \text{ vertical forces} = 0$$

so

$$\Sigma 100 + 400 - 600 - R + 4000 = 0$$

thus R $= 3900$ N
This is beyond the measure of force that will cause small fractures in the cartilaginous plates at the vertebral disc junction. It is clearly much too high to correspond with a reasonably moderate activity like shovelling in a flexed posture. While the figures in this example are open to criticism, being partly chosen for simplicity rather than accuracy, more sophisticated calculations arrive at similar conclusions. Various mechanisms have been suggested that act to relieve the compression forces on discs and vertebrae.

The contribution of the posterior ligaments and the way their passive stretch to different degrees may help to resist flexion forces has been noted in Chapter 11. It is further suggested that the posterior ligaments are able to distribute tension generated by backward rotation of the pelvis up to the thoracic spine. It must be remembered that bending of the whole trunk is being resisted and the concept (presented in Fig. 2.8) of tension on the stretching aspect and compression on the shortening aspect is relevant. Thus, the more tension generated in the posterior structures – posterior ligaments and erector spinae muscles – the larger the area in which compression acts and so the lower the stress (force) per unit area. The elasticity of the posterior ligaments in standing has already been noted. This means that they are prestressed so that the spine acts like a prestressed beam (see Chapter 2). Further tensing of the posterior ligamentous structures can be produced, it is suggested, by a pull on the thoracolumbar fascia when the transversus abdominis contracts. The deep and superficial layers of the posterior laminae of the thoracolumbar fascia are composed of fibres passing not only laterally but angled to each other so that pulling on them tends to approximate their attachments at the vertebral spines, see Fig. 12.3. Another suggestion is that, as the thoracolumbar fascia envelops the erector spinae muscle, pulling on it increases the pressure within this tubular fascial sheath thus increasing its resistance to being flexed (Norris, 1995). It is also argued that the lumbar facet joints and their capsules are significant in resisting compression between individual vertebrae.

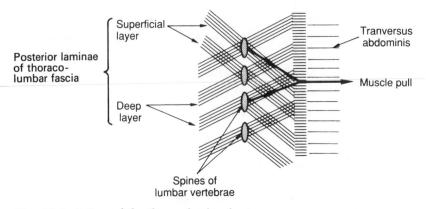

Fig. 12.3 Action of the thoracolumbar fascia.

RANGE OF MOTION OF THE SPINE

Movements of the spine depend on the motion of the individual vertebrae on one another. there is considerable variation in both the total spinal motion and, to a lesser extent, the pattern of individual segmental motion. However, some general features are reasonably consistent. About half the flexion and extension evident in the cervical region is due to movement at the atlanto-occipital joint, the rest occurring in the joints found between the second and seventh cervical vertebrae, mostly in the lower two cervical joints. As would be expected, all movements are rather limited in the thoracic region due to the arrangement of the ribs. Flexion and extension are usually considered to be limited to about 5° between each pair of vertebrae for the upper three-quarters of this region. The lower thoracic segments have rather more motion, merging into the markedly greater sagittal motion, of some 75°, of the five lumbar vertebral joints.

Side flexion is fairly consistent, being about 5° to each side in the cervical region and lower thoracic segments, but rather less, 3° or so, in the intervertebral joints in most of the thoracic and lumbar regions. Rotation of 4° or 5° to each side occurs in the cervical and upper two-thirds of the thoracic region, but is very limited in the lower thoracic and lumbar regions. The large range of rotation possible to each side (90° or so) in the cervical region is allowed by the free range of rotation that occurs at the atlantoaxial joint. While separate rotation and side bending can be performed in all regions, it should be noted that these movements are normally combined. The degree of movement allowed between vertebrae depends on the vertical thickness of the intervertebral disc in relation to its area. Thus, cervical and lumbar discs are relatively thick to allow the greater movement of these regions. The direction of movement is constrained by the orientation of the facet joints and the movements permitted at the costovertebral joints.

THE HIP JOINT

The hip joint is a synovial ball and socket joint between the concave acetabulum of the pelvis and the convex head of the femur. It bears very large forces in locomotion and yet has considerable mobility. Both surfaces are covered by articular cartilage, thicker in the regions that are in contact in the standing position. The acetabular socket is deepened by the fibrocartilaginous labrum and the joint is stabilized by extremely strong capsular ligaments.

Ranges of motion of the hip

In the sagittal plane, the hip has a total range of flexion and extension of some 140°, a total in the coronal plane of abduction and adduction of about 80°, and a total rotation in the horizontal plane of about 90° (based on figures from the American Academy of Orthopedic Surgeons, 1965). As described in Chapter 9, only a small proportion of this total range is utilized during walking. Flexion in the sagittal plane is maximum during the latter part of the swing phase, being about 30–35° beyond the neutral position in standing. At heel off the hip is at its most extended, being about 5–10° beyond neutral (see Fig. 9.6). The hip joint will also move in the coronal plane, abducting and adducting as the pelvis tilts at each step. Rotation will also occur at each step as each side of the pelvis moves alternately forward, as described in Chapter 9. The range of these two motions has been found in normal men to average 12° and 13° respectively (Johnston and Smidt, 1969). It should be noted, once again, that such figures are averages and, while the walking cycles of a single individual are usually highly consistent, others differ considerably from one another. Further, the velocity of the gait dictates the ranges of motion, larger ranges being associated with higher velocities. Age alters the pattern to some extent in that step length tends to shorten in old age, so a smaller range of hip motion is needed.

Table 12.2 Mean measurements of maximum hip motion in various activities

Activity	Sagittal (flex + ext) (°)	Coronal (abd + add) (°)	Horizontal (med + lat rot) (°)
Tying shoelaces with foot on floor	124	19	15
Tying shoelaces with foot across opposite thigh	110	23	33
Sitting down and rising from chair	104	20	17
Squatting	122	28	20
Walking up stairs	67	16	18

The range of hip motion in normal men in three planes during everyday activities has been measured with an electrogoniometer (Johnston and Smidt, 1970). Some examples are given in Table 12.2. It will be seen that a considerable range of hip motion is needed for bending down, tying a shoelace and squatting, whereas climbing stairs involves relatively little range of motion. Even less flexion and extension are needed in descending stairs.

Forces at the hip

Standing on both feet in a normal upright position places the centre of gravity of the body approximately half way between the two hip joints. Thus, the joint reaction force on the head of the femur – the force pressing femur and acetabulum together – is about one-third of the body weight. (Each lower limb is about one-sixth of the body weight (see Chapter 3) and the remaining two-thirds is equally divided between the two hips.) Some muscle action is likely to stabilize the trunk on the hips and this will add compression between the surfaces, so the force is actually rather more. If the weight is taken on only one lower limb the situation is very different. The line of gravity must pass through the standing foot and medial to the hip joint. How far it lies from the hip depends on the posture of the rest of the body. It will be closest when the upper trunk is sideflexed well over the standing hip. In other postures it will be much more medial (Frankel and Nordin, 1980). The pelvis is therefore a horizontal first order lever pivoted at the hip, the body weight being counterbalanced by contraction of the hip abductor muscles holding the lateral end down on to the femur (see Fig. 12.4). Since, in standing, the system is in equilibrium, the moments of force acting on this lever must add to zero. The distances of both the line of gravity (length 'a' in Fig. 12.4) and abductor muscle attachment from the axis of the hip ('b' in Fig. 12.4) can be measured radiographically or estimated with reasonable accuracy on a standing subject; the body weight can then be measured. The muscle force of the abductors (M) can be found from:

$$\Sigma (W \times \text{distance from axis}) - (M \times \text{distance from axis}) = 0$$

Reasonable figures for the distances a and b in an adult might be 10 cm and 5 cm respectively. W is five-sixths of the body weight, the standing leg being approximately one-sixth of body weight. Therefore:

$$\Sigma (W \times 10) - (M \times 5) = 0$$

thus, $M = 2W = 1.66$ of body weight.

The term 'abductor muscles' has been used to mean the gluteus medius, minimus and tensor fasciae latae. All of these are considered to contribute to stabilizing the pelvis but in differing proportions; the ratios of their

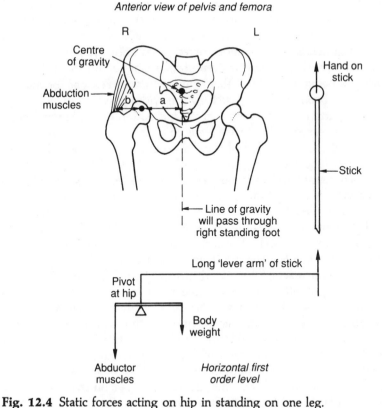

Anterior view of pelvis and femora

Fig. 12.4 Static forces acting on hip in standing on one leg.

masses were found to be gluteus medius 4, gluteus minimus 2 and tensor fasciae latae 1 (Inman, 1947). Due to their differing attachments around the hip, their contribution will vary with the position of the joint. In any case, the total force they exert in standing on one leg must be greater than 1.66 of body weight derived above because they are all at some acute angle to the horizontal so that only a part of their pull acts at right angles to the pelvic lever (see Chapter 5). (In some positions, tensor fasciae latae may be at a right angle.)

The joint reaction force in the hip is found from these forces by simple addition of vertical forces, thus:

$$\Sigma W + (1.66 \times W) - R = 0$$

where R is the reaction force at the hip and will, therefore, in this example, be 2.21 body weight.

Thus, the force at the hip joint can be seen to be high when standing on one leg. More detailed calculations give an average figure of around 2.75 times body weight for the static position. During locomotion, the figure will be much higher at times because the body weight is being accelerated upwards at each step. During each step, there are two peaks: one at heel strike and one just prior to toe off (see Chapter 9). The load on the hip in men has been described (Frankel and Nordin, 1980) as around four times body weight at heel strike and about seven times body weight just before toe off. In women, the pattern was reported as similar, but the magnitude was much less being around half that of men. Various reasons for this sex difference have been advanced, such as the wider pelvis coupled with a different gait pattern, or differences in the inclination of the femoral neck, for example. Increased gait velocity leads to further increases in this force.

It is clear that the magnitude of the joint reaction force depends on the ratios of the distances between the line of gravity to the axis of the hip and the attachment of abductor muscles to this axis. As noted already, the line of gravity will depend on upper body and pelvic positions. In circumstances in which the abductors are weakened (by paralysis or altered alignment, as occurs in congenital dislocation of the hip) the 'gravity lever arm' is shortened at each step by sideflexing the trunk over the stance leg to give the typical 'Trendelenburg gait'. This same action minimizes the joint reaction force and this gait is thus adopted by those with painful degenerative arthritis. Some relief in both circumstances is achieved by the use of a stick in the opposite hand. This allows the opposite arm to help to shift the pelvis over the supporting hip, thus reducing the contraction needed in the abductors. While the force that can be exerted by the arm on the stick is relatively small, the effect is considerable because of the length of the lever. This idea is represented in Figure 12.4. It is suggested that this reduces the load on the leg by 60% (Goldie and Dumbleton, 1981). This effect leads to the well known paradox in stick usage, when an elderly patient, using a stick in one hand for balance, fractures the femoral neck on this same side. During rehabilitation, the stick is used in the opposite hand to allow the weight to be relieved from the healing femur as well as aiding balance. Subsequent recovery allows the stick to be returned to the original side, as it is being used for balance only. Surgical intervention can also alter the ratios between the abductor muscle and gravitational levers. If the greater trochanter is moved laterally, for example, it increases the length of the muscle lever to lower joint reaction forces. Similarly, varus osteotomy, by moving the femur medially, diminishes the joint load (Goldie and Dumbleton, 1981).

While the hip joint reaction force is very variable and can be quite high, this is not necessarily undesirable in normal subjects. Calculations and measurements indicate this marked variation; standing on one leg has been shown to lead to forces 2.4–2.6 times the body weight (Inman, 1947). Forces ranging from 2.3 times body weight for a slowly walking woman to 5.8 for a man walking energetically, and a variation from 1.3 to 5 times body weight in going from slow walking to running, have been found by others. Nonetheless the pain of degenerative arthritis of the hip is increased by loading the joint and reduced by unloading, as occurs in the sideflexing gait. Some theoretical calculations of hip joint loading have been made (Murray and Gore, 1981). Based on a man of body weight 82.4 kg (70 kg when the weight of the standing leg, at 15% of body weight, is subtracted), the joint load is calculated at 210 kg or about 2.5 times the body weight. When repeating the calculations on assuming that the patient's weight has increased by 10 kg, the joint load is increased by 30 kg to nearly 2.8 times the body weight. The deleterious effects of such patients being significantly overweight are obvious. The effect of a lurching (Trendelenburg) gait was calculated assuming that the lever length of the line of gravity ('a' on Fig. 12.4) could be reduced from 10 cm to 3 cm. This provided a marked reduction in joint load to 112 kg, or just 1.3 times the body weight. The effect of holding a stick in the opposite hand 40 cm from the loaded hip and applying 14 kg to the stick (thought not to be unreasonable) decreased the joint load to 84 kg, which is close to body weight. While these figures are theoretical, there is some experimental support for the reduction of abductor activity and hence of reduced joint loading. While the gait alterations of sideflexing and using a stick appear to be highly beneficial to those patients with a painful hip, it must be recognized that, in both cases, there is some increased energy cost. The sideflexion of the lurching Trendelenburg gait means that the centre of gravity of the body must oscillate from side to side with a greater amplitude. Since the kinetic energy is proportional to the square of the velocity (kinetic energy $= \frac{1}{2}mv^2$) and the velocity will increase in proportion to the amplitude of the motion, such lurching will lead to markedly increased energy usage. If the centre of gravity oscillates with twice the normal amplitude, it will need about four times as much energy (Murray and Gore, 1981). While the additional energy necessary for the use of a stick in the opposite hand is difficult to calculate, it is likely to be considerably less than that of the abnormal gait to achieve the same benefit in reduced joint loading.

THE NECK OF THE FEMUR

As described in the section on the hip joint, the forces applied to the femoral head in all locomotive activities are very great. They are transmitted between the shaft and head of the bone through the narrow angled neck. The stresses generated in the internal bony structure of the neck are therefore considerable, since both body weight and the abductor muscle forces are transmitted.

The angle of inclination between the axis of the shaft and the axis of the neck of the femur in the coronal plane is about 125° in the adult, having decreased from 150° in the newborn (Singleton and LeVeau, 1975). It can be seen that the weight of the supported body acting through the head of the femur will produce both shear stress and a bending stress. The bending stress will produce compression forces on the medial side of the femoral neck and tensile stress on the lateral side. However, during weightbearing, the hip abductors contract forcibly, which tends to

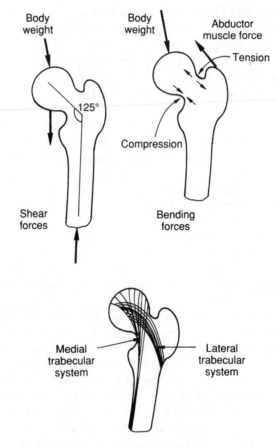

Section of upper femur

Fig. 12.5 Stresses on the femoral neck and trabecular patterns.

counteract the tension stress on the lateral side of the neck. The point was noted in Chapter 2, in which the greater toleration in bone of compression forces over tension or shear stresses was noted. These points are illustrated in Figure 12.5.

Bone tissue develops structure according to the stresses to which it is subjected. The bony trabeculae of the upper end of the femur form a pattern that is similar in overall plan, although individuals differ in the detail. As might be expected, the greatest bone density occurs where the greatest stress is developed. Two major trabeculae systems have been identified.

The medial system arises from the cortical bone of the medial side of the shaft, passes up the medial side of the neck towards the centre of the head from where it fans outwards to the articular surface of the head. This group is near-vertical in direction (about 79° with the horizontal) and seems to be aligned with the direction of joint force that occurs in one-legged stance. It would thus seem to be developed to resist these compression forces (Singleton and LeVeau, 1975).

A lateral system formed from the dense cortical bone on the lateral side of the shaft and base of the greater trochanter passes upwards and medially, lying on the lateral side of the neck to the centre of the head. The line of its trabeculae crosses those of the medial system at an angle (see Fig. 12.5). It is considered by some that this system acts mainly to resist compression due to the abductor muscle action. However, this is not universally agreed, as there is some evidence that it has a more important role in resisting tensile forces. There is, of course, no dispute that this system will resist both tension and compression, but only which of these is its principal purpose.

It will be noted that the trabeculae from these two systems, crossing as they do, form a series of arches, which spread the load on the femoral head to the dense cortical bone of the shaft. A third plate of denser trabeculae called the 'calcar femorale' runs up from the dense bone of the linea aspera to the posterior wall of the neck and great trochanter.

These trabecular patterns are most evident in a coronal plane but actually exist in a three-dimensional arrangement, which is much more complicated.

The upper femoral epiphysis lies almost at right angles to the medial trabecular system, thus placing it in a position of least shearing stress but maximum compression. It is suggested that a slipped upper femoral epiphysis – a condition that occurs mainly in pubescent boys – occurs partly as a result of large shear forces. This is supported by the fact that the majority of these patients are obese, which causes larger than normal forces on the femur (Chung and Hirata, 1981).

THE KNEE

This is the largest joint in the body and sustains remarkably high forces, being both a weightbearing joint and responsible for joining the two longest rigid bony levers of the body. The tibiofemoral joint is a double condylar articulation with rounded femoral condyles separated from the flatter tibial surface by two menisci. The patellofemoral joint is sellar and a functional part of the knee joint. Inspection of these bones suggests that the knee lacks stability but this erroneous assumption is corrected when the size and strength of the ligamentous and muscular tissues involved is appreciated. The close-packed position of the joint is in full extension, when all the ligaments are in a tightened position. The cruciate ligaments act to prevent sliding of the surfaces; the anterior cruciate prevents the tibia slipping forwards on the femur and the posterior ligament prohibits backward sliding. In other positions of the joint, the ligaments are a little slack to allow both rotation and trivial lateral motion, but at least one of the cruciate ligaments is taut in all positions acting firmly to unite tibia and femur.

The major movements of the knee are flexion and extension in a range of about 150°, from some 5° beyond the vertical (hyperextension) to 140–160° of flexion, which is limited by contact of the calf on the posterior thigh tissues. The shape of the femoral condyles dictates that the axis of this movement will move upwards and forwards during knee extension, and backwards and downwards during flexion. The movement consists of both rolling and sliding, and takes place between the femoral condyles as one surface and the menisci with the tibia moving as the other. If the tibia is fixed (as occurs with the foot on the ground), the femur rotates medially during the last 30° or so of extension. This is often called the 'screw home' movement or 'locking' mechanism, since it leads to spiral tensing of the ligaments and, ultimately, the fully close-packed position. The cause of this rotary motion, which occurs around a near-vertical axis through the lateral condyle, has been ascribed to mechanisms involving both the shapes of the articular surfaces and ligamentous and muscular tension. As the knee approaches full extension, the lateral femoral condyle reaches its fully extended position before the medial condyle, causing the femur to rotate medially as extension continues. Although starting to occur about 30° before full knee extension, this rotation is most evident and occurs most rapidly in the last few degrees of extension. It is called 'conjunct rotation', as it is an inevitable part of the natural joint motion, as opposed to 'adjunct rotation', which occurs in the knee as a result of muscle action or external forces. The range of conjunct rotation during flexion and extension is about 20°. If the tibia is being extended on a relatively fixed femur, the same process occurs but it is, of course, the tibia that rolls and slides forwards, rotating laterally near full extension. Note that the femur rolls forwards but slides backwards (see 'The shape and motion of synovial joints', pp. 218–219). In flexion, the reverse process occurs. It is believed that contraction of the popliteus muscle initiates the lateral rotation (of the femur) that occurs in flexion and pulls back the posterior part of the lateral meniscus.

Rotation – adjunct rotation – is greatest when the knee is in 90° of flexion, reducing with either further flexion or extension. In the close-packed, fully extended position it is obviously zero. At 90° of flexion, some 70° of total rotation is possible, more than half being lateral rotation from the neutral position. This movement occurs between the tibia and menisci with the femoral condyles. A few degrees of abduction and adduction are possible in the semiflexed knee, about 10° in total.

Due to the length of the limb segments involved, flexion and extension at the knee is an obviously large visible motion, whereas the rotation is barely evident. This leads to the importance of rotary motion being disregarded, yet it exhibits a range of motion of nearly half the total range of sagittal motion, and, as indicated, normal flexion and extension is impossible without it. The fact that the joint is divided by the menisci into two compartments, in which the two distinct movements occur, adds to the significance of independent rotation at the knee.

For many functional activities, the knee moves in a sagittal plane, approximately through a right angle from full extension (see Table 12.3).

Table 12.3 Range of sagittal motion at the knee

Activity	Angle of flexion from full extension (°)
Climbing stairs	83
Descending stairs	90
Sitting down	93
Bending down to tie shoelaces	106
Full squat	160

Modified from Frankel and Nordin, 1980.

In normal walking, the joint passes through a sagittal range of just under 70°. Full extension is unusual so that the joint is in about 5° of flexion both at heel strike and just prior to toe off, increasing to about 70° near the middle of the swing phase (Murray *et al.*, 1964). Conjunct rotation of about 10° or so on average appears to occur during the gait cycle, lateral rotation occurring, as would be expected, during knee extension and medial rotation during flexion in the swing phase. A small amount of abduction occurs during extension and adduction during flexion in the walking cycle. As described in Chapter 9, the knee flexes during walking in order to shorten the forward swinging leg, so that, in climbing slopes or walking over irregular ground, the gait pattern alters to one with greater knee flexion. Furthermore, during the stance phase, the knee appears to be less fully extended the faster the gait. The range of knee flexion from full extension for a variety of activities is shown in Table 12.3. These figures may be compared with those for sagittal motion at the hip joint given in Table 12.2, since these two motions are mutually dependent in such activities.

The patella slides on the femoral condyles during flexion and extension of the joint through a distance of about 7 cm in the adult. In the range in which most functional movement occurs, from full extension to 90°, both femoral condyles are in contact with the posterior articular surface of the patella, which has two matching surfaces. Near full knee flexion the most medial facet on the patella is in contact with the medial femoral condyle.

Magnitude of joint reaction forces at the knee

As described in the section on the hip joint, the forces at the joint surfaces – the joint reaction forces – are likely to vary markedly during the gait cycle or other moderate activity and be several times the body weight at their peaks. The maximum reaction forces occurring during the cycle are associated with muscle contractions stabilizing the knee. Thus, following heel strike, a reaction force of two to three times the body weight occurs, due to contractions of the hamstring muscles. In the early stance phase, a joint reaction force of about double the body weight

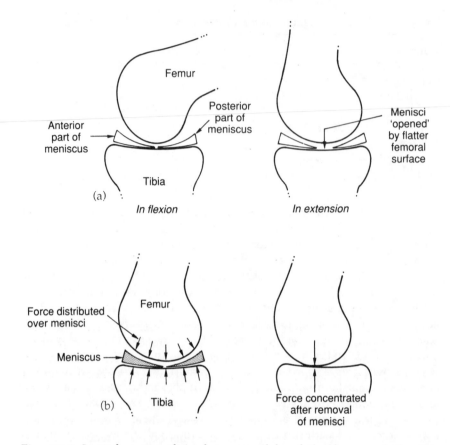

Fig. 12.6 Sagittal section through one condyle of the femur and the tibia showing relationship of the menisci.

occurs in association with the quadriceps contraction needed to prevent the knee flexing too far. Just before toe off, another peak develops due to contraction of the gastrocnemius; this could be up to four times the body weight, but has been found to be variable between subjects (Morrison, 1970). In general, the higher reaction forces of the stance phase seem to be borne more by the larger medial tibial surface with its thicker articular cartilage than by the lateral surface. The tension forces acting on the knee ligaments in walking are much lower than the compressive joint reaction forces; the posterior cruciate is considered to sustain the highest forces to about half body weight (Morrison, 1970).

Purposes of the menisci

The semilunar fibrocartilages partly separate the femoral from the tibial condyles. It has been noted above that they allow the two movements of

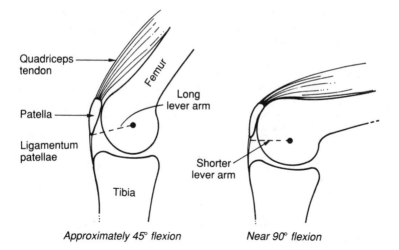

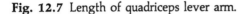

Fig. 12.7 Length of quadriceps lever arm.

the knee to occur separately on either surface, a feature common to joints divided by articular discs. They also help to support the joint reaction forces, making the femoral and tibial articular surfaces more nearly congruent (see Fig. 12.6). As the flatter parts of the femoral condyles contact the menisci during extension of the knee, so the curve of the menisci is opened, allowing a matching, flatter tibiomeniscal-bearing surface (see Fig. 12.6a). If the menisci are surgically removed, the area in which contact between the femur and the tibia occurs is reduced leading to higher local stresses (see Fig. 12.6b). A further function of the menisci is considered to be a role in lubrication. The articular damage that is found to occur following prolonged vigorous exercise of the knee after meniscectomy may be the result of the increased local stress or the loss of lubricating efficiency, or both. The menisci normally regenerate from their periphery after meniscectomy.

The patellofemoral joint

The patella is the largest sesamoid bone in the body, being developed in the tendon of the quadriceps. It serves to provide a rigid, relatively large bearing surface as the tendon passes over the bending joint. This increased area of contact between the tendon and the femur allows a better distribution of stress, thus reducing compression. It also lengthens the lever arm of the quadriceps by increasing the distance of the tendon from the axis of rotation in the femoral condyles (Fig. 12.7). This is not a uniform increase throughout the range of motion because of the shape of the patella and the surface of the femoral condyles on which it moves. At about 45° of flexion, the effect is greatest but, nearer to full extension, the distance is reduced somewhat. During flexion from 45°, the patella sinks deeper between the femoral condyles so that the lever arm is at its shortest. This is shown in Table 12.4 and Figure 12.7.

Table 12.4 Quadriceps moment arm

Knee joint angle (°)	Quadriceps moment arm (cm)
Full extension	
5	4.4
45	4.9
60	4.7
90	3.8
Full flexion	

Data based on Smidt, 1973.

While this arrangement allows greater force to be provided by the quadriceps to straighten the knee, it is not the only purpose of the patella. It is true that, if the patella is surgically removed, the quadriceps tendon runs closer to the axis of the joint, meaning that greater force must be exerted by the quadriceps to straighten the knee. However, during knee extension, the patella is being pulled upwards by the quadriceps but it is also forced forwards by the shape of the femoral condyles, so that the ligamentum patellae and the attached tibia move a greater distance than the quadriceps tendon. This gives a faster movement of the tibia but with less force. The patella is not merely a part of the 'rope' of a simple pulley system but serves to alter the line of pull (see Alexander, 1992, for a clear explanation).

Walking involves relatively little flexion of the knee and low forces generated in the quadriceps, as noted above. It is not surprising, then, that the joint reaction force between the patella and the femur is relatively low. In fact, the highest values during the walking cycle — at about the middle of the stance phase when loaded knee flexion was at its maximum — has been calculated to be about half the body weight (Reilly and Martens, 1972). In situations where body weight is being moved on a more flexed knee, at knee flexion of around 90°, the patellofemoral joint reaction force has been found to be very much greater, at about three times the body weight. In general, the reaction force increases with greater knee flexion, apparently increasing more rapidly after about 60°. It is recognized that patients suffering from degenerative disorders of the patellofemoral articulation experience more pain in semiflexion than near full extension of the knee, which conforms with these mechanical findings. There is a striking difference in this pattern of joint reaction forces if the resistance to knee extension is provided by some force other than body weight. If resistance is provided by a weight at the foot — a deLorme boot, for

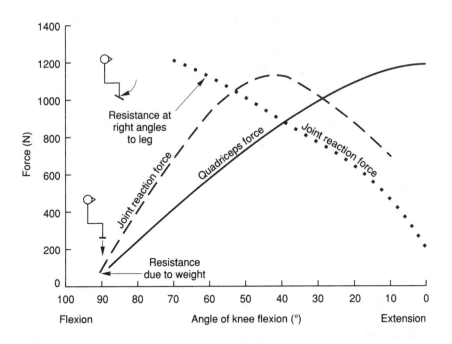

Fig. 12.8 Patellofemoral joint reaction forces and muscle force of quadriceps against angle of knee extension (modified from Frankel and Nordin, 1980).

example – with the free-hanging leg moving from 90° flexion to full extension, then the force is zero at first, but rises rapidly to a peak then diminishes again towards full extension (see Fig. 12.8). If manual, or some other resistance, is given at right angles to the leg, the joint reaction force is at maximum in 90° of flexion and diminishes towards full extension. In both cases, the quadriceps force was least at 90°, increasing steadily to a maximum at full knee extension (see also Chapter 5). These points are illustrated in Figure 12.8. This explains why quadriceps exercises are able to be performed comfortably in a small range near full extension by patients with some patellofemoral derangements, but often provoke pain if performed with greater flexion of the knee.

THE FOOT

Foot support, mobility and stability

The foot acts to support the body weight. The area of the under surface of the foot in contact with the ground can easily be investigated by taking footprints (a wet foot on absorbent paper, for example) or by directly inspecting the whitened pressure areas in an angled mirror below a strong glass plate on which the subject stands. In relaxed standing, the areas of

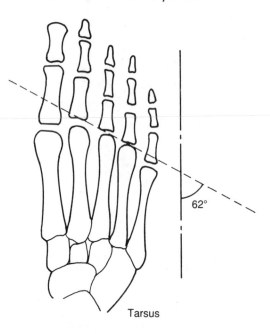

Tarsus

Fig. 12.9 Common axis of motion of metatarsophalangeal joints at push off.

contact are the heel (calcaneum) and the forefoot (metatarsal heads, especially the first), and a variable area along the lateral border of the foot. The principal contact areas can also be recognized by the skin thickening that occurs. The mid-part of the foot and much of the medial border is rarely in contact with the ground due to the general arched structure.

While standing on both feet, the muscles acting on and within the foot are largely quiescent, so that the downward force of the body weight, which would tend to deform the foot by spreading the arch, is resisted by ligaments. If the load on the foot is increased by standing on one foot, it will be found that the area of contact increases. This has the effect of both diminishing the increase in pressure that would otherwise occur and making balancing easier. The feet of young children are relatively large, which is also an aid to balance in the early stages of walking. Whereas the lengths of the femur and the tibia take until the age of three years to reach half their adult length, the foot reaches this size in about one year in girls and one and a half in boys (Frankel and Nordin, 1980).

Rising onto the toes brings all the weight on to the metatarsal heads. At the same time, the calcanei invert and the whole foot becomes near-rigid. Thus, the foot changes from a weightbearing structure to a rigid lever able to transmit force from the attachment of the tendo calcaneus to the metatarsal heads without bending. This change, from a flatter weight-supporting structure to a rigid arched lever, occurs in walking. As the heel rises at heel off, the toes are passively dorsiflexed at the metatarso-phalangeal joints. Much of the weight taken through the forefoot during

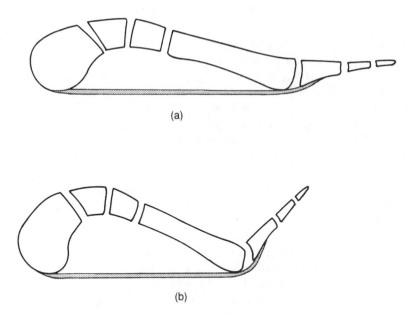

(a)

(b)

Fig. 12.10 The action of the plantar fascia in producing a rigid arched foot: (a) arch flat and metatarsophalangeal joints straight; (b) arch raised by dorsiflexion at the metatarsophalangeal joints pulling on the plantar fascia.

the stance phase passes through the head of the first metatarsal and, as the heel rises, the weight distribution shifts laterally. At push-off, the five metatarsophalangeal joints are dorsiflexed in a line joining their average centres of rotation. This line is at an angle to the long axis of the foot (see Fig. 12.9). The position of this line is clearly evident in the crease lines of well worn shoes. It forms an average angle of 62° with the long axis of the foot, but varies with individuals by some 10° either way (Inman *et al.*, 1981).

The way in which the arch of the foot is stabilized for walking and, more significantly, for running and jumping, is complex. The numerous intertarsal and tarsometatarsal joints allow only restricted individual movement because of their irregular and interlocking joint surfaces, as well as their strong ligamentous connections, but collectively the movement is considerable. They can be held in a near extreme position – fully arched foot – by both muscle action and fascial tension. The muscles involved include both the intrinsic foot muscles and some leg muscles, notably the tibialis posterior, which attaches to almost all the tarsal bones and the peroneus longus. The plantar fascia acts like a truss across the longitudinal arch of the foot. When the metatarsophalangeal joints are passively dorsiflexed while rising on the toes, the largely inextensible plantar fascia is pulled across these joints to shorten and reduce the distance between metatarsal heads and the calcaneous (see Fig. 12.10).

THE FIRST METATARSOPHALANGEAL JOINT

The big toe makes an important and unique contribution to locomotion. It is the final point of contact with the ground in toe off and provides final push-off in both fast walking and running, as discussed in Chapter 9. The head of the first metatarsal is involved in weightbearing during standing – on average, one-sixth of the weight supported by the foot (Frankel and Nordin, 1980) – and to a much greater degree in walking and running. The weight is actually distributed via two sesamoid bones in the tendons of flexor hallucis brevis, which lie in the grooves on the under surface of the convex metatarsal head.

The movements allowed at this joint are flexion, extension, abduction and adduction. Of these, extension, at about 90°, is significant, the rest allowing only a few degrees of motion. This is the functional movement needed for the locomotor role of this joint.

Two features are striking about the muscles acting over this joint. One is the size, and hence the strength, of the flexor hallucis longus muscle, and the other is the large number of muscle pulls that can act on the phalanges of the big toe. The clear purpose is stabilization and exact control of the position of this joint. Thus, the flexor hallucis longus acts to press the phalanges downwards on to the ground and yet prevent hyperextension. The sesamoid bones are controlled not only by the tendons of flexor hallucis brevis, in which they lie, but also on the medial side by the large abductor hallucis and on the lateral side by the two heads of adductor hallucis pulling at different angles. While the abductor and the adductor have their named action, they are both sited near the plantar aspect of the joint, suggesting their importance in control while the joint is extended.

THE SHOULDER GIRDLE AND SHOULDER JOINT COMPLEX

The structures uniting the upper limb to the trunk are complicated and serve to allow the hand an extremely wide range of motion. Changing the position of the arm involves movement of the humerus, clavicle and scapula at the glenohumeral, acromioclavicular and sternoclavicular joints as well as the gliding of the scapula over the thoracic wall. Furthermore, there are numerous bursae to facilitate motion between adjacent structures, in particular the subacromial and subscapular bursae.

The sternoclavicular joint is a synovial joint between the larger medial end of the clavicle and a somewhat smaller facet on the manubrium. The joint cavity is totally divided by a fibrocartilaginous, intra-articular disc, which is attached above to the upper part of the medial end of the clavicle and below to the first costal cartilage (see Fig. 12.11a). The joint is stabilized by a strong capsule and ligaments, but the principal structures securing the clavicle are the disc and the strong costoclavicular ligament. This latter is formed of the two laminae uniting the inferior surface of the clavicle to the first rib and its cartilage, the anterior layer passing upwards and laterally

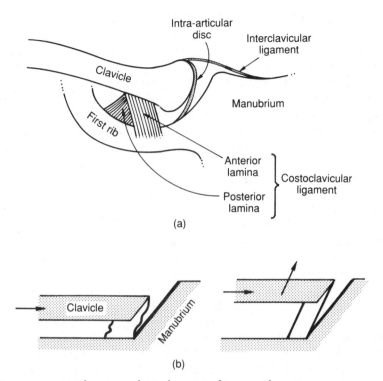

Fig. 12.11 (a) The sternoclavicular joint; (b) coronal section.

and the posterior upwards and medially (Fig. 12.11a). The movements that are allowed consist of elevation and depression of the lateral end of the clavicle, which occurs between the clavicle and the disc, and protraction and retraction, mainly between the disc and the manubrium. The axes for both these movements lie close to the costoclavicular ligament. A certain amount (about 40°) of rotation around the long axis of the clavicle is allowed and occurs mainly during arm elevation. The two parts of the costoclavicular ligament may act separately to limit the two extremes of this rotation (Williams *et al.*, 1989). It can be seen from the coronal section of the joint shown in Figure 12.11a that forces applied to the arm or shoulder and tending to drive the clavicle medially will cause it to ride up the manubrial surface. This movement would be strongly resisted by tensing of both the costoclavicular ligament and the disc (Fig. 12.11b).

The acromioclavicular joint is a synovial joint between a small oval convex facet on the lateral end of the clavicle and a similar concave facet on the medial border of the acromion. The joint cavity is partly divided by an intra-articular disc. The capsule and the superiorly sited acromioclavicular ligament contribute to stability, but the most important structure uniting the bones, and thus stabilizing the joint, is the coracoclavicular ligament. The anterolateral trapezoid part of this ligament passes laterally from the coracoid, almost horizontally to the inferior surface of the

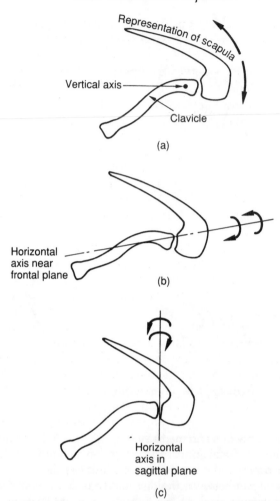

Fig. 12.12 Movements of acromioclavicular joint (representation of scapula and clavicle seen from above): (a) anteroposterior movement of scapula as in protraction and retraction; (b) rotation of the scapula so that the inferior angle swings from the resting position upwards, forwards and laterally or upwards, backwards and medially around the chest wall; (c) scapula moving so that inferior angle moves laterally away from the chest wall and back (based on Frankel and Nordin, 1980).

clavicle above. The anatomically and functionally separate conoid part of the ligament is almost vertical, attaching the conoid tubercle on the inferior clavicular surface to an area at the root (medial edge) of the coracoid process. Both parts serve to keep the clavicle and the coracoid process closely approximated, so closely that in some subjects the presence of bursae and cartilage form a coracoclavicular joint (Williams *et al.*, 1989). The ligament thus limits the upward movement of the clavicle. Elevation of the arm leads to the scapula rotating and moving the coracoid process away from the clavicle pulling on the conoid ligament. This pulls the most posterior part of the S-shaped clavicle downwards, causing it to rotate backwards in its long axis. This rotation, of about 40–50° at maximum, allows full elevation of the upper limb. If clavicular rotation is prevented, active abduction is limited to 120° (Peat, 1986). (In this function, the movement of the clavicle can be likened to that of a crank, in which movement of the off-set part causes rotation of the main shaft.) At the acromioclavicular joint, the joint surfaces are angled in the coronal plane such that, when they are pressed together, as in a fall on the outstretched arm, the acromion tends to push under the clavicle, forcing it upwards. The trapezoid ligament is believed to be the principal prevention to overriding (Peat, 1986). The mechanism is identical to that described for the sternoclavicular joint and costoclavicular ligament, as illustrated in Figure 12.11b.

Movement at the acromioclavicular joint can occur in three planes. First, the scapula can move forwards and backwards in protraction and retraction of the shoulder, so that the acromion glides forwards and backwards on the meniscus and the clavicle, around the vertical axis of the conoid ligament. Secondly, the scapula can hinge (around the trapezoid ligament), moving around an axis that is in an approximately frontal (coronal) and horizontal plane. The scapula is thus moving approximately around the long axis of the clavicle in the plane of its own body. This movement occurs between the meniscus and the clavicle. Thirdly, the scapula can move a little around a horizontal axis in the sagittal plane, the whole scapula moving in a coronal plane. These movements are illustrated in Figure 12.12. While the ranges of motion of the various acromioclavicular movements are small (some 20–30° is often cited), coupled with the somewhat greater sternoclavicular motion, they allow considerable shoulder girdle movement, as described later.

The glenohumeral joint is a synovial, multiaxial ball and socket joint, with the rounded articular surface of the humeral head much larger than the pear-shaped glenoid fossa. The head is some three or four times larger and the joint surfaces are not congruous, except in the close-packed position of abduction and lateral rotation. The glenoid articular cavity is enlarged and its edges are protected by the flexible fibrocartilaginous labrum, which may also assist in lubrication of the joint. The tendons of the long heads of biceps brachii and triceps are attached and reinforce this labrum. The capsule is relatively thin and loose but is reinforced by ligaments and muscle attachments. The coracohumeral ligament is important in resisting the downward pull on the shoulder joint in the relaxed and dependent arm, as described below. The stability of the joint is greatly dependent on the contribution of the short muscles, whose attachments are blended intimately with the capsule. Anteriorly, the subscapularis, superiorly the supraspinatus, and posteriorly the infraspinatus and teres minor, are collectively called the rotator cuff. It will be noted that these muscles form a horseshoe around the joint, leaving the inferior aspect not supported in this way, but to some degree upheld by the tendon of the long head of

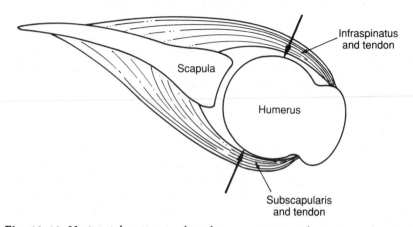

Fig. 12.13 Horizontal section to show how contraction of anterior and posterior muscles may push the head of the humerus to help to stabilize it.

triceps. (Since this is clearly not a cuff, why the name? Apparently, it is derived from the anglicization or mistranslation of the French 'coiffe' literally a 'head-dress' and implying here the horseshoe-shaped plait of hair worn on the top of the head by some women.) The effects of these four muscles on the movement and stability of the joint are extremely important. It should be noted that the fibres of these muscles converge on the capsule from the extensive area of both sides of the whole body of the scapula. They are (except teres minor) essentially triangular muscles, whose fibres converge on to a small area from a range of angles, which allows force to be exerted in many directions to control movement of the humeral head. Furthermore, as the head of the humerus is so much larger than the glenoid, these muscles are wrapped around the head in a horizontal plane, as illustrated in Figure 12.13. Their contraction will not only approximate their attachments but also press on the humeral head. Thus, the subscapularis will not only effect medial rotation of the humerus but will also cause the head to slide backwards on the glenoid. Similarly, the actions of the posteriorly placed muscles will cause lateral rotation and forward sliding (Frankel and Nordin, 1980).

Scapulothoracic mechanism

The concave surface of the scapula moves over the thoracic wall during shoulder girdle motion. The subscapularis fascia moves on the serratus anterior and thoracic wall; a little loose areolar tissue in this space allows motion. The serratus anterior, attached to the vertebral border of the scapula, is important in holding the scapula in close contact with the thoracic wall. It has been suggested, without supporting evidence, that the bulging of these two muscles when they are contracted may help stabilize the scapula.

Movements of the humerus, scapula and clavicle

The movements that can occur at the multiple joints just described are inevitably complex. Essentially, the glenoid provides a platform on which the rounded head of the humerus can move in an infinite variety of planes. The platform itself can be moved up, down, forwards and backwards, and rotated by scapular movement to give an even greater range of motion. In describing motion at these joints, it is best to consider motion of the humerus in respect to the scapula rather than in relation to the axes and planes of the anatomical standing position. Thus, abduction of the arm is described 'in the plane of the scapula'. In the normal standing posture, the body of the scapula lies in a plane between 30° and 45° anterior to the coronal (or frontal) plane. In describing these complex movements, it is important to recognize that wide variations occur not only between individuals but also in the same individual when moving the limb with different loads. Even the position from which the movement starts varies. It has been found that, with the arm hanging near vertically at the side, the angle of the scapula can vary by as much as 20°.

If the arm is moved from the side of the body through abduction to full elevation, the first 30° or so is almost entirely glenohumeral motion. Subsequently, scapular and glenohumeral motion occur together, with motion at the sternoclavicular joint of about 40° and a further 20° at the acromioclavicular joint. The remainder is motion at the glenohumeral joint. Inspection of the movement of arm elevation will show that in many subjects the scapula actually makes a minor movement at the very onset of arm motion. This is considered to be due to muscles stabilizing the scapula in a suitable position preparatory to movement of the humerus. At about 30° of abduction, the scapula and clavicle together start to rotate about an imaginary axis through the clavicle (near the sternoclavicular joint) to the root of the spine of the scapula (Fig. 12.14a); elevation of the clavicle on the disc at the sternoclavicular joint occurring, as described above. Once the costoclavicular ligament becomes taut, upward clavicular motion is halted, at about 100° of elevation, so that further scapular rotation occurs at the acromioclavicular joint about horizontal axes in near frontal and sagittal planes (see Figs 12.12 and 12.14b). As full elevation is approached, tension in the coracoclavicular ligament imposes backwards rotation on the clavicle, as described above, to allow further upward rotation of the glenoid cavity. About two-thirds of the movement of elevation can be ascribed to the glenohumeral joint alone, the rest occurring as scapular motion. This 2 : 1 ratio is not universally agreed, as several researchers have found very different ratios: anything from 1.25 : 1 to 2.3 : 1. Apart from the individual differences to be expected, it seems that elevation in different planes and with different loads may lead to a different pattern. It has been found that heavier loads on the arm lead to earlier scapular motion. Impairment of glenohumeral movement due to injury or disease – supraspinatus tendinitis, for example – leads to an alteration in elevation due to inhibition of the glenohumeral contribution.

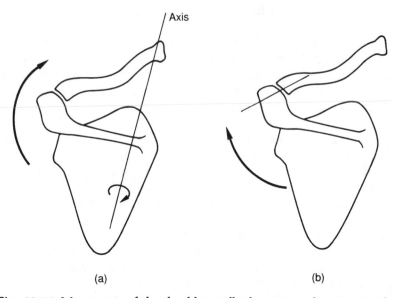

(a)   (b)

Fig. 12.14 Movements of the shoulder girdle during arm elevation: (a) clavicle and scapula rotate together, moving at sternoclavicular joint; (b) scapula rotates further, moving at acromioclavicular joint.

Excessive early scapular movement on attempted arm abduction is referred to as an abnormal 'scapulohumeral rhythm'.

During elevation, the humerus also rotates laterally about its long axis. This is necessary in order to prevent impingement of the greater tuberosity on the acromion process.

In passing, it may be noted that elevation of the arm in upward reaching activities is associated with postural changes in the trunk. Although full elevation is normally described as occurring through 180° at the shoulder, many subjects exhibit an increased lumbar lordosis in the later stages of bilateral elevation to reach the vertical arm position. In unilateral arm elevation, an even more evident side flexion of the trunk occurs. This not only serves to increase the vertical reach by raising one shoulder but can be seen to occur in many activities, in overarm throwing, for example.

Static stability of the shoulder joint

During natural standing, the relaxed arm hangs vertically at the side and the weight of the arm would be expected to slide the head of the humerus downwards on the glenoid. At one time it was suggested that activity in the deltoid and other muscles in the long axis of the arm gave support, but there is no detectable activity in these muscles. The support is actually due to tension of the upper part of the capsule, the coracohumeral ligament and, sometimes, activity in supraspinatus and the posterior fibres of the

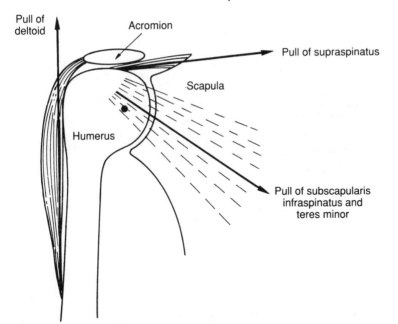

Fig. 12.15 The muscle forces causing abduction of the humerus.

deltoid. The way this can work is due to the obliquity of the glenoid fossa, which faces forwards, laterally and a little upwards in the normal standing posture. Downward sliding of the humeral head causes it to move laterally because of the obliquity of the glenoid, thus tensing the upper fibres of the capsule and coracohumeral ligament. Supraspinatus also acts in this way (Basmajian, 1974). In principle, the mechanism is the same as that illustrated by Figure 12.11b; Figure 12.15 also shows this. It is suggested that the frequent occurrence of glenohumeral subluxation in hemiplegic patients is due to the relative abduction allowed at the joint because of the drooping shoulder girdle, which prevents the operation of this locking mechanism (Basmajian, 1974).

The support of the whole shoulder girdle in the normal standing position must be provided principally by tension in the upper fibres of trapezius and levator scapulae muscles. It was believed at one time that low level activity was needed in these muscles to maintain this posture, but it has been found (Bearn, 1961) that there is no electromyographic activity in most people and surprisingly little even when the arm is loaded. This demonstrates the effectiveness of the normal elasticity of musculotendinous and other collagenous tissue. Some contribution may also be made by the rhomboids and the upper part of serratus anterior.

Abduction at the glenohumeral joint

This movement is essentially performed by contraction of the deltoid in

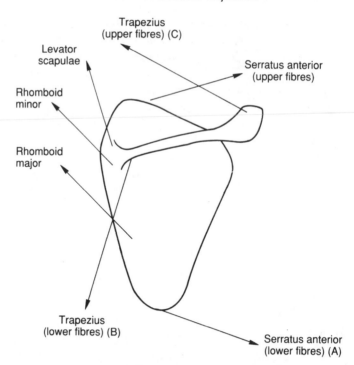

Fig. 12.16 Muscles connecting the scapula to the trunk. Note that when A, B and C contract simultaneously, lateral rotation occurs. Note also that A has a long lever arm for rotation about the root of the spine and about the acromioclavicular joint.

conjunction with the rotator cuff muscles. With the arm at the side, the pull of the deltoid is largely upward with a small lateral component acting below the axis of movement. The subscapularis, infraspinatus and teres minor pull downward and medially above the axis. The supraspinatus pulls medially above the axis (see Fig. 12.15). The result is a strong force couple turning the limb through abduction. As the straight arm abducts to 90°, the force needed rises to a maximum but diminishes in further elevation. The joint reaction force at 90° has been variously calculated to be anything from 50% to 90% of body weight (Peat, 1986). The long head of biceps brachii can also make a contribution in helping to stabilize the humeral head against upward sliding. When the arm is laterally rotated, this tendon, with its attachment to the supraglenoid tubercle and running in the bicipital groove, can act like a pulley rope and assist abduction.

Control of the scapula

Apart from the upper fibres of trapezius and the pectoralis minor, all the muscles uniting the scapula to the trunk are attached close to the medial border. The stoutness of this part and of the spine of the scapula indicate the strong forces applied. The general direction of the pull of the muscles is shown in Figure 12.16. This illustrates how the scapula is stabilized in all directions. Lateral rotation of the scapula, when the arm is elevated, is provided by co-contraction of the lower fibres of serratus anterior of trapezius, and of the upper fibres of trapezius, which forms a strong force couple. These serve to turn the scapula about an axis through the root of the spine and about the acromioclavicular joint.

Appendix A:
Power of 10 notation

This is a method of making the handling of large numbers much simpler. Basically it obviates the need to read and write long strings of noughts and allows multiplication and division to be done by addition and subtraction, which is much easier. It is also known as scientific notation. The basis is set out in Table A.1. The small superscript number to the right of the 10 is called the exponent.

Table A.1 Power of 10 notation

10^{-4}	0.0001	one-ten-thousandth
10^{-3}	0.001	one-thousandth
10^{-2}	0.01	one-hundredth
10^{-1}	0.1	one-tenth
10^{0}	1	one
10^{1}	10	ten
10^{2}	100	a hundred
10^{3}	1000	a thousand
10^{4}	10 000	ten thousand
10^{5}	100 000	a hundred thousand
10^{6}	1 000 000	a million
10^{7}	10 000 000	ten million
10^{8}	100 000 000	a hundred million
10^{9}	1 000 000 000	a billion*

*Almost universally, the word billion refers to 1 000 000 000 (one thousand million) or 10^{9}. Formerly in the UK the word meant 1 000 000 000 000 (one million million) or 10^{12}. In the USA, and increasingly in the UK, this is referred to as a trillion.

Notice that in Table A.1 the numbers have sensible meanings. Thus 10 squared (10^{2}) is 100 and similarly the negative powers are *reciprocals* of the numbers, so that $10^{-2} = 1/100 = 0.01$. Notice also that the power of 10 notation is much shorter to write than the equivalent numerical or word representation for all but the shortest positive numbers. The larger the number, the more convenient the system becomes – Table A.1 could be extended both upwards (negative) and downwards (positive).

The value of any given power of 10 notation can be found in another way by considering the exponent to indicate the location of the decimal point. After putting down the initial 1, the place of the decimal point is determined by the number of noughts given by the exponent, to the right for positive and the left for negative (Table A.2).

So far the power of 10 notation has been considered only with regard to 10, 100, 1000 and so forth, but any number can be described by the system. When 10^2 is written it is the same as 1×10^2 and means 100.

Table A.2 Power of 10 notation

−4	−3	−2	−1	0	1	2	3	4
↓	↓	↓	↓	↓	↓	↓	↓	↓
0	0	0	0	0	0	0	0	0

So:

10^{-4}	move decimal point 4 places to left of 1 =	0.0001
10^{-3}	move decimal point 3 places to left of 1 =	0.001
10^{-2}	move decimal point 2 places to left of 1 =	0.01
10^{-1}	move decimal point 1 place to left of 1 =	0.1
10	move decimal point 0 places from 1 =	1
10^{1}	move decimal point 1 place to right of 1 =	10
10^{2}	move decimal point 2 places to right of 1 =	100
10^{3}	move decimal point 3 places to right of 1 =	1000
10^{4}	move decimal point 4 places to right of 1 =	10 000

Similarly, 2×10^2 would be 200 and 2.4×10^2 would be 240. In this way any number can be written as the digit or digits times some power of 10.

What has been described up to this point is a convenient method of describing numbers but the real value and strength of the notion lie in the ability to simplify calculations. In order to multiply two numbers together, all that is necessary is to add the exponents, for example;

$$10^2 \times 10^3 \ (100 \times 1000) = 10^5 \ (100\,000) \text{ because} + 2 + 3 = 5$$
$$10^2 \times 10^{-4} \ (100 \times 0.0001) = 10^{-2} \ (0.01) \text{ because} + 2 - 4 = -2$$
$$10^2 \times 10^{-2} \ (100 \times 0.01) = 10^0 \ (1) \text{ because} + 2 - 2 = 0$$

This explains why 10 can be taken as 1.

In the same way, division of numbers can be effected by subtracting the exponents, for example:

$$\frac{10^4}{10^2} = \frac{10000}{100} = 10^2 \ (100)$$
$$(\text{because} + 4 - 2 = +2)$$

or

$$\frac{10^{-1}}{10^2} = \frac{0.1}{100} = 10^{-3} \ (0.001)$$
$$(\text{because} - 1 - 2 = -3)$$

Appendix B:
Trigonometric ratios

In a triangle with one right angle, the ratio of the lengths of the sides are proportional to the angles. The sides may be named:

Hypotenuse: the side opposite the right angle;
The side opposite the angle of interest;
The side adjacent to the angle of interest.

The sine (sin) of an angle is the ratio of the side opposite to the hypotenuse, thus:

$$\sin = \frac{\text{length of side opposite}}{\text{length of hypotenuse}}$$

For example, sine 30° = 0.5, meaning that the side opposite is half the length of the hypotenuse.

Similarly, the cosine (cos) of an angle is given by:

$$\cos = \frac{\text{length of side adjacent}}{\text{length of hypotenuse}}$$

For example, cosine 30° = 0.866, meaning that the adjacent side is 86.6% of the length of the hypotenuse.

The ratio of side opposite and side adjacent is called the tangent (tan) of the angle:

$$\tan = \frac{\text{length of side opposite}}{\text{length of side adjacent}}$$

For example, tan 30° = 0.577.

The sines, cosines and tangents are given for all angles in sets of tables and stored in scientific calculators, so that knowledge of the angle and the length of one side allows calculation of the other sides. If the length is proportional to, say, a force, then the other force can be found. If the values of all the forces are unknown, then the proportion of the force acting in a particular direction may be calculated; see Figure 1.3b for an example.

References

CHAPTER 1

Nigg B.M. (1994) Selected historical highlights. In: Nigg B.M. and Herzog W. (eds.) *Biomechanics of the Musculo-skeletal System.* pp. 3–35. Wiley, Chichester.

Ritchie-Calder (Lord). (1970) Conversion to the metric system. *Scientific American,* **223**, 17–25.

CHAPTER 2

Alexander R.M. (1992) *The Human Machine.* Natural History Museum Publications, London.

Cromer A.H. (1981) *Physics for the Life Sciences,* 2nd edn. McGraw-Hill, New York.

Frankel V.H. and Burstein A.H. (1970) *Orthopaedic Biomechanics.* Lea and Febiger, Philadelphia.

Frankel V.H. and Nordin M. (1980) *Basic Biomechanics of the Skeletal System.* Lea and Febiger, Philadelphia.

Gordon J.E. (1978) *Structures: or Why Things Don't Fall Down.* Penguin Books, London.

Halbertsma J.P.K. and Göeben L.N.H. (1994) Stretching exercises: effect on passive extensibility and stiffness in short hamstrings of healthy subjects. *Archives of Physical Medicine and Rehabilitation,* **75**, 976–981.

Kazarian L.E. and von Gierke H.E. (1969) Bone loss as a result of immobilisation and chelation. Preliminary results in Macaca Mulatta. *Clinical Orthopaedics,* **65**, 67–75.

Noyes F.R. (1977) Functional properties of knee ligaments and alterations induced by immobilisation. *Clinical Orthopaedics,* **123**, 210–242.

Noyes F.R. and Grood E.S. (1976) The strength of the anterior cruciate ligament in humans and Rhesus monkeys. Age-related and species-related changes. *Journal of Bone and Joint Surgery* (Boston, MA), **58A**, 1074–1082.

Radin E.L., Rose R.M., Blaha J.D. *et al.* (1992) *Practical Biomechanics for the Orthopaedic Surgeon,* 2nd edn. Churchill Livingstone, Edinburgh.

Reilly D. and Burstein A.H. (1975) The elastic and ultimate properties of compact bone tissue. *Journal of Biomechanics,* **8**, 393–405.

Rutherford O.M. (1990) The role of exercise in prevention of osteoporosis. *Physiotherapy,* **76**, 522–526.

CHAPTER 3

Alexander R.M. (1992) *The Human Machine.* Natural History Museum Publications, London.

Cody K.A. and Nelson A.J. (1978) The effect of vertical perception on body balance in normal subjects. *Physical Therapy,* **58**, 35–41.

Gabell A. and Simons M.A. (1982) Balance coding. *Physiotherapy,* **68**, 286–288.

Grandjean E. (1980) *Fitting the Task to the Man: An Ergonomic Approach.* Taylor and Francis, London.

The Health of the Nation: A strategy for health in England. (1992) White paper. HMSO. London.

Karpovich P.V. (1959) *The Physiology of Muscular Activity,* 5th edn. Saunders, Philadelphia.

Lane R.E. (1969) Physiotherapy in the treatment of balance problems. *Physiotherapy,* **55**, 415–420.

Reilly T. and Secher N. (1990) Physiology of sport: an overview. In: Reilly T., Secher N., Snell P. and Williams C. (eds.) *Physiology of Sports.* E. and F.N. Spon (an imprint of Chapman and Hall), London.

Sheldon W.H., Stevens E.S. and Tucker W.R. (1940) *The Variation of Human Physique.* Harper, New York.

Shipman P. (1994) Those ears were made for walking. *New Scientist,* (July), 26–29.

US Department of Health, Education and Welfare. (1966) *Weight, Height and Selected Body Dimensions of Adults: United States 1960–62.* (Vital and Health Statistics, series II, no. 8) Government Printing Office, Washington.

Williams M. and Lissner H.R. (1962) *Biomechanics in Human Motion.* Saunders, Philadelphia.

CHAPTER 4

Berger R.A. (1982) *Applied Exercise Physiology.* Lea and Febiger, Philadelphia.

Buller A.J. (1973) Posture and movement. *Physiotherapy,* **59**, 344–349.

Clamann H.P. (1993) Motor unit recruitment and the gradation of muscle force. *Physical Therapy,* **73**, 830–843.

Gowitzke B.A. and Milner M. (1980) *Understanding the Bases of Human Movement,* 2nd edn. Williams and Wilkins, Baltimore.

Lieber R.L. and Bodine-Fowler S. (1993) Skeletal muscle mechanics: implications for rehabilitation. *Physical Therapy,* **73**, 844–856.

Reilly J., Secher, N., Snell P. *et al.* (1990) *Physiology of Sports.* Chapman and Hall, London.

Salmons S. and Vbrova C. (1969) The influence of activity on some contractile characteristics of mammalian fast and slow muscles. *Journal of Physiology,* **210**, 535–549.

Williams P. L., Warwick R., Dyson M. *et al.* (1989) *Gray's Anatomy,* 37th edn. Churchill Livingstone, Edinburgh.

CHAPTER 5

Berger R.A. (1982) *Applied Exercise Physiology*. Lea and Febiger, Philadelphia.

Bickers M.J. (1993) Does verbal encouragement work? The effect of verbal encouragement on a muscular endurance task. *Clinical Rehabilitation*, **7**, 196–200.

de Lorme T.L. and Watkins A.L. (1957) *Progressive Resistance Exercise: Technic and Medical Application*. Appleton-Century-Crofts, New York.

Edwards R.H.T., Young A., Hosking G.P. and Jones D.A. (1977) Human skeletal muscle function: description of tests and normal values. *Clinical Science and Molecular Medicine*, **52**, 283–290.

Grandjean E. (1980) *Fitting the Task to the Man: an Ergonomic Approach*. Taylor and Francis, London.

Holder-Powell H.M. and Jones D.A. (1990) Fatigue and muscular activity: a review. *Physiotherapy*, **76**, 672–679.

Howe T.E. and Oldham J.A. (1995) Reliability of measuring quadriceps cross-sectional area with compound B ultrasound scanning. *Physiotherapy*, **81**, 241.

Hyde S.A., Scott O.M. and Goddard C.M. (1983) The myometer: the development of a clinical tool. *Physiotherapy*, **69**, 424–427.

Lieber R.L. and Bodine-Fowler S.C. (1993) Skeletal muscle mechanics: implications for rehabilitation. *Physical Therapy*, **73**, 844–856.

MacConaill M.A. (1949) Movements of bones and joints; function of musculature. *Journal of Bone and Joint Surgery (Br)*, **31B**, 100–104.

Mayhew T.P. and Rothstein J.M. (1985) Measurement of muscle performance with instruments. In: Rothstein J.M. (ed.) *Measurement in Physical Therapy*. Churchill Livingstone, New York, 57–102.

Moritani T. (1993) Neuromuscular adaptations during the acquisition of muscle strength, power and motor tasks. *Journal of Biomechanics*, **26**, Suppl I, 95–107.

Peacock B., Westers T., Walsh S. and Nicholson K. (1981) Feedback and maximum voluntary contraction. *Ergonomics*, **3**, 223–228.

Prilutsky B.I. and Zatsiorsky V.M. (1994) Tendon action of two-joint muscles: transfer of mechanical energy between joints during jumping, landing and running. *Journal of Biomechanics*, **27**, 25–34.

Williams M. and Lissner H.R. (1962) *Biomechanics of Human Motion*. Saunders, Philadelphia.

Young A. and Hughes I. (1982) Ultrasonography of muscles in physiotherapeutic practice and research. *Physiotherapy*, **69**, 187–190.

Zajac F.E. (1993) Muscle co-ordination of movement; a perspective. *Journal of Biomechanics*, **26** (Suppl I), 109–124.

CHAPTER 6

Alexander R.M. (1992) *Exploring Biomechanics: Animals in Motion*. Scientific American Library, New York.

American Academy of Orthopedic Surgeons. (1965) *Joint Motion: a Method of Measuring and Recording*. Chicago.

Basic Biomechanics Explained

Beighton P., Grahame R. and Bird H. (1983) *Hypermobility of Joints.* Springer-Verlag, Berlin.

Boone D.C., Azen S.P., Lin C-M. *et al.* (1978) Reliability of goniometric measurements. *Physical Therapy,* **58**, 1358–1360.

Coutts F., Hewetson D. and Matthews J. (1989) Continuous passive motion of the knee joint: use at the National Orthopaedic Hospital, Stanmore. *Physiotherapy,* **75**, 427–431.

Davies S.P. (1991) Effect of continuous passive movement and plaster of Paris after internal fixation of ankle fractures. *Physiotherapy,* **77**, 516–520.

Dumbleton J.H. and Black J. (1981) Principles of mechanics. In: Black J. and Dumbleton J.H. (eds.) *Clinical Biomechanics: a Case History Approach.* Churchill Livingstone, New York.

Gajdosik R.L. and Bohannon R.W. (1987) Clinical measurement of range of motion. *Physical Therapy,* **67**, 1867–1872.

Harms M. and Engstrom B. (1991) Continuous passive motion as an adjunct to treatment in physiotherapy management of the total knee arthroplasty patient. *Physiotherapy,* **77**, 301–307.

Hellebrandt F.A., Duvall E.N. and Moore M.I. (1949) The measurement of joint motion, Part III: Reliability of goniometry. *Physical Therapy Review,* **29**, 302–307.

Low J.L. (1963) A simple method of measuring shoulder elevation. *Physiotherapy,* **49**, 214.

Low J.L. (1976a) The reliability of joint measurement. *Physiotherapy,* **62**, 227–229.

Low J.L. (1976b) Measurement of joint motion. *New Zealand Journal of Physiotherapy,* **5**, 23–29.

Metcalf V.A. and Yeabel M.A. (1972) Documentation of hand function with the use of office copying equipment. *Physical Therapy,* **52**, 535–538.

Nicol A.C. (1989) Measurement of joint motion. *Clinical Rehabilitation,* **3**, 1–8.

Norkin C.C. and White D.J. (1985) *Measurement of Joint Motion: a Guide to Goniometry.* Davies, Philadelphia.

Rose M.J. (1991) The statistical analysis of the intra-observer repeatability of four clinical measurement techniques. *Physiotherapy,* **77**, 89–91.

Williams M. and Lissner H. R. (1962) *Biomechanics of Human Motion.* Saunders, Philadelphia.

Wright V. (1973) Stiffness: a review of its management and physiological importance. *Physiotherapy,* **59**, 107–111.

Youdas J.W., Carey J.R., Garrett T.R. *et al.* (1994) Reliability of goniometric measurements of active arm elevation in the scapular plane obtained in a clinical setting. *Archives of Physical Medicine and Rehabilitation,* **75**, 1137–1144.

CHAPTER 7

Alexander R.M. (1992) *The Human Machine.* Natural History Museum Publications, London.

Cromer A.H. (1981) *Physics for Life Sciences.* McGraw Hill, Auckland.

Davis B.C. and Harrison R.A. (1988) *Hydrotherapy in Practice.* Churchill

Livingstone, Edinburgh.

Golland A. (1981) Basic hydrotherapy. *Physiotherapy,* **67**, 258–262.

Hall J., Bisson D. and O'Hare P. (1990) The physiology of immersion. *Physiotherapy,* **75**, 517–521.

Harrison R.A. and Bulstrode S. (1987) Percentage weight bearing during partial immersion in the hydrotherapy pool. *Physiotherapy Practice,* **3**, 60–63.

Harrison R.A., Hillman M. and Bulstrode S. (1992) Loading of the lower limb when walking partially immersed: implications for clinical practice. *Physiotherapy,* **78**, 164–166.

Hillman M.R., Matthews L. and Pope J.M. (1987) The resistance to motion through water of hydrotherapy table-tennis bats. *Physiotherapy,* **33**, 570–572.

Martin J. (1981) The Halliwick method. *Physiotherapy,* **67**, 288–295.

Reid Campion M.J. (1990) *Adult Hydrotherapy.* Butterworth-Heinemann, Oxford.

Skinner A.T. and Thompson A.M. (1983) *Duffield's Exercise in Water,* 3rd edn. Baillière Tindall, London.

Skinner A.J. and Thompson A.M. (1994) Hydrotherapy. In: Wells P.E., Frampton V. and Bowsher D. (eds.) *Pain: Management by Physiotherapy,* 2nd edn. Butterworth-Heinemann, Oxford.

Tovin B.J., Wolf S.L., Greenfield B.H. *et al.* (1994) Comparison of the effects of exercise on water and on land on the rehabilitation of patients with intra-articular anterior cruciate ligament reconstruction. *Physical Therapy,* **74**, 710–719.

CHAPTER 8

Clark W.B., Prescott P.R., McGregor A.B. *et al.* (1974) Pneumatic compression of the calf and post-operative deep vein thrombosis. *Lancet,* **ii**, 5–7.

George P.A. (1975) Compression treatment for hypertrophic scars. *Physiotherapy,* **51**, 215–216.

Gillham L. (1994) Lymphoedema and physiotherapeutics: control not cure. *Physiotherapy,* **80**, 835–843.

Gray R. (1987) The management of limb oedema in patients with advanced cancer. *Physiotherapy,* **73**, 504–506.

Hills N. H., Phlug J. J., Jeyasingh K. *et al.* (1972) Prevention of deep vein thrombosis by intermittent pneumatic compression of the calf. *British Medical Journal,* **i**, 131–135.

Knight M.T.N. and Dawson R. (1976) Effect of intermittent compression of the arms on deep vein thrombosis in the legs. *Lancet,* **ii**, 1265–1268.

Rithalia R.V.S., Sayegh A. and Edwards J. (1987) Concurrent report on intermittent compression devices. *Clinical Rehabilitation,* **1**, 65–70.

Salter M. (1987) *Hand Injuries: a Therapeutic Approach.* Churchill Livingstone, Edinburgh.

Sayegh A., Rithalia R.V.S. and Andrews K. (1987) Performance characteristics of intermittent pneumatic compression systems. *Clinical Rehabilitation,* **1**, 71–75.

Thomas S., Dawes C. and Hay P. (1981) A critical evaluation of some extensible bandages in current use. *New Zealand Journal of Physiotherapy,* **9**, 23–26.

CHAPTER 9

Alexander R.M. (1992) *The Human Machine.* Natural History Museum Publications, London.

Beheshti Z. (1994) Biodynamic basis of rhythmic limb movement in humans. *Physiotherapy*, **80**, 599–603.

Butler P.B. and Major R.E. (1992) The learning of motor control: biomechanical considerations. *Physiotherapy*, **78**, 6–11.

Dyson G. (1968) *The Mechanics of Athletics.* University of London Press, London.

Gardiner M.D. (1981) *The Principles of Exercise Therapy*, 4th edn. Bell and Hyman, London.

Gillis B., Gilroy K., Lawley H. *et al.* (1986) Slow walking speeds in healthy young and elderly females. *Physiotherapy Canada*, **38**, 350–352.

Hageman P.A. and Blanke D.J. (1986) Comparison of gait of young women and elderly women. *Physical Therapy*, **66**, 1382–1387.

Halkberg G. (1976) A system for the description and classification of movement behaviour. *Ergonomics*, **19**, 727–739.

Harrison K. and Jackson J. (1994) Relationships between mental practice and motor performance. *British Journal of Therapy and Rehabilitation*, **1**, 14–18.

Inman V.T., Ralston H.J. and Todd F. (1981) *Human Walking.* Williams and Wilkins, Baltimore.

Joseph J. (1964) The activity of some muscles in locomotion. *Physiotherapy*, **50**, 180–183.

Marteniuk T.G. (1979) Motor skill performance: considerations for rehabilitations. *Physiotherapy Canada*, **78**, 6–11.

McGuiness-Scott J. (1982) Benesh movement notation: an introduction to recording clinical data. *Physiotherapy*, **68**, 182–184.

Murray M.P., Drought A.B. and Kory R.C. (1964) Walking patterns of normal men. *American Journal of Bone and Joint Surgery*, **46A**, 335–359.

Murray M.P., Kory R.C. and Clarkson B.H. (1969) Walking patterns in healthy old men. *Journal of Gerontology*, **24**, 169–178.

Sloman L., Berridge M., Homatidis S. *et al.* (1982) Gait patterns of depressed patients and normal subjects. *American Journal of Psychiatry*, **139**, 94–97.

Smidt G.L. (1990) *Gait in Rehabilitation (Clinics in Physical Therapy).* Churchill Livingstone, New York.

Whittle M. (1991) *Gait Analysis: an Introduction.* Butterworth-Heinemann, Oxford.

CHAPTER 10

Berger R.A. (1982) *Applied Exercise Physiology.* Lea and Febiger, Philadelphia.

The Health of the Nation: A strategy for health in England. (1992) White paper. HMSO. London.

Karpovich P.V. (1959) *Physiology of Muscular Activity*, 5th edn. Saunders, Philadelphia.

MacGregor J. (1981) The evaluation of patient performance using long term ambulatory monitoring technique in the domiciliary environment.

Physiotherapy, **67**, 30–33.

Saradeth, T., Ernst, E. and Darburger, L. (1991) The kinetics of exercise leucocytes. *European Journal of Physical Medicine and Rehabilitation*, **2**, 44–49.

Sharp C. and Parry-Billings M. (1992) Can exercise damage your health. *New Scientist*, (15 Aug), 33–37.

Waters R. and Yakura J. (1990) Energy expenditure of normal and abnormal ambulation. In: Smidt G.L. (ed.) *Gait in Rehabilitation*. Churchill Livingstone, Edinburgh, 65–96.

Whittle M. (1991) *Gait Analysis: an Introduction*. Butterworth-Heinemann, Oxford.

CHAPTER 11

Andersson B.J.G. and Ortengren R. (1974) Lumbar disc pressure and myoelectric back muscle activity during sitting. *Scandinavian Journal of Rehabilitation Medicine*, **3**, 115–121.

Basmajian J.V. (1974) *Muscle Alive*, 3rd edn. Williams and Wilkins, Baltimore.

Burton R.F. (1994) *Physiology by Numbers*. Cambridge University Press, Cambridge.

Corlett E.N., Hutcherson C., DeLugan M.A. *et al.* (1972) Ramps or stairs: the choice using physiological and biomechanical criteria. *Applied Ergonomics*, **3**, 195–201.

Dul J. and Weerdmeester B. (1991) *Ergonomics for Beginners: a Quick Reference Guide*. Taylor and Francis, London. (First published in English, 1993.)

Foster M. (1988) Ergonomics and the physiotherapist. *Physiotherapy*, **74**, 484–489.

Frankel V.H. and Nordin M. (1980) *Basic Biomechanics of the Skeletal System*. Lea and Febiger, Philadelphia.

Grandjean E. (1985) *Fitting the Task to the Man*. Taylor and Francis, London.

Health and Safety Executive. (1992a) *Manual Handling Operations Regulations*. HMSO, London.

Health and Safety Executive. (1992b) *Guidance on Manual Handling of Loads in the Health Service*. HMSO, London.

Irvine C.H., Snook S.H. and Sparshatt J.H. (1990) Stairway risers and treads: acceptable and preferred dimensions. *Applied Ergonomics*, **21**, 215–225.

Jackson S. (1995) An investigation of the claims made about balance chairs. *Physiotherapy*, **18**, 451.

Jensen G.M. (1980) Biomechanics of the lumbar intervertebral disk; a review. *Physical Therapy*, **60**, 765–773.

Kroemer K.H.E. (1964) Heute Zutreffende Körpermasse. *Arbeitswissenschaft*, **3**, 42–45.

Livingstone L.A., Stevenson J.M. and Olney S.J. (1991) Stair climbing kinematics on stairs of differing dimensions. *Archives of Physical Medicine and Rehabilitation*, **72**, 398–402.

Mandel A.C. (1976) Workchair with tilting seat. *Ergonomics*, **19**, 157–164.

Mortimer R.G. (1974) Foot brake pedal force capability of drivers. *Ergonomics*, **17**, 509–513.

Nachemson A.L. (1960) Lumbar intradiscal pressure. *Acta Orthopaedica Scandinavica Supplementum*, **43**, 104–140.

Nachemson A.L. (1976) The lumbar spine: an orthopaedic challenge. *Spine*, **1**, 59–71.

Nachemson A.L. and Evans J.H. (1968) Some mechanical properties of the third human lumbar interlaminar ligament (ligamentum flavum). *Journal of Biomechanics*, **1**, 211–220.

National Institute for Occupational Safety and Health. (1981) *Work Practices Guide for Manual Lifting*. NIOSH, Cincinnati.

Oborne D.J. (1995) *Ergonomics at Work*. Wiley, Chichester.

Radin E.L., Blaha J.D., Rose R.M. *et al.* (1992) *Practical Biomechanics for the Orthopaedic Surgeon*, 2nd edn. Churchill Livingstone, Edinburgh.

Smith A.G., Orpwood R.D. and Palmer M. (1984) A controllable-rise chair. *Physiotherapy*, **70**, 265.

CHAPTER 12

Alexander R.M. (1992) *The Human Machine*. Natural History Museum Publications, London.

American Academy of Orthopedic Surgeons (1965) *Joint Motion: A Method of Measuring and Recording*. Chicago.

Basmajian J.V. (1974) *Muscles Alive*, 3rd edn. Williams and Wilkins, Baltimore.

Bearn J.G. (1961) An electromyographic study of the trapezius, deltoid, pectoralis major, biceps and triceps muscles during static loading of the upper limb. *Anatomical Record*, **140**, 103–108.

Chung S.M.K. and Hirata T.T. (1981) Multiple pin repair of the slipped capital femoral epiphysis. In: Black J. and Dumbleton J.H. (eds.) *Clinical Biomechanics: a Case History Approach*. Churchill Livingstone, Edinburgh, 94–115.

Frankel V.H. and Nordin M. (1980) *Basic Biomechanics of the Skeletal System*. Lea and Febiger, Philadelphia.

Goldie I.F. and Dumbleton J.H. (1981) Intertrochanteric osteotomy of the femur. In: Black J. and Dumbleton J.H. (eds.) *Clinical Biomechanics: a Case History Approach*. Churchill Livingstone, Edinburgh, 72–93.

Gordon J.E. (1978) *Structures: or Why Things Don't Fall Down*. Penguin Books, London.

Inman V.T. (1947) The functional aspects of the abductor muscles of the hip *American Journal of Bone and Joint Surgery*, **29**, 607–619.

Inman V.T., Ralston H.J. and Todd F. (1981) *Human Walking*. Williams and Wilkins, Baltimore.

Johnston R.C. and Smidt G.L. (1969) Measurements of hip joint motion during walking. Evaluation of an electrogoniometric method. *Journal of Bone and Joint Surgery* (Am), **51A**, 1083–1085.

Johnston R.C. and Smidt G.L. (1970) Hip motion measurements for selected activities of daily living. *Clinical Orthopaedics*, **72**, 205–208.

McNeil T.W. (1981) The role of spine fusion in the treatment of problems of the lumbar spine. In: Black J. and Dumbleton J.H. (eds.) *Clinical Biomechanics: a Case*

History Approach. Churchill Livingstone, Edinburgh, 317–334.

Morrison J.B. (1970) The mechanics of the knee joint in relation to normal walking. *Journal of Biomechanics,* **3,** 51–61.

Murray M.P., Drought A.B. and Kory R.C. (1964) Walking patterns of normal men. *American Journal of Bone and Joint Surgery,* **46A,** 335–359.

Murray M.P. and Gore D.R. (1981) Gait of patients with hip pain or loss of hip joint motion. In: Black J. and Dumbleton J.H. (eds.) *Clinical Biomechanics: a Case History Approach.* Churchill Livingstone, Edinburgh, 173–200.

Norris C.M. (1995) Spinal stabilisation: 3. Stabilisation of the lumbar spine. *Physiotherapy,* **81,** 72–79.

Peat M. (1986) Functional anatomy of the shoulder complex. *Physical Therapy,* **66,** 1855–1865.

Radin E.L., Rose R.M., Blaha J.D. *et al.* (1992) *Practical Biomechanics for the Orthopaedic Surgeon.* Churchill Livingstone, Edinburgh.

Reilly D.T. and Martens M. (1972) Experimental analysis of the quadriceps muscle force and patello-femoral joint reaction force in various activities. *Acta Orthopaedica Scandinavica,* **43,** 126–137.

Singleton M.C. and LeVeau B.F. (1975) The hip joint: structure, stability and stress. *Physical Therapy,* **59,** 957–972.

Smidt G.L. (1973) Biomechanical analysis of knee flexion and extension. *Journal of Biomechanics,* **6,** 79–92.

Williams P.L., Warwick R., Dyson M. *et al.* (1989) *Gray's Anatomy,* 37th edn. Churchill Livingstone, Edinburgh.

Index

Index